SYMPOSIA OF THE SECTION ON MICROBIOLOGY

THE NEW YORK ACADEMY OF MEDICINE

Number 8

CELLULAR METABOLISM
AND INFECTIONS

CELLULAR METABOLISM
AND INFECTIONS

EDITED BY

E. Racker

SYMPOSIUM HELD AT THE

NEW YORK ACADEMY OF MEDICINE

MARCH 4 AND 5, 1954

1954   New York

ACADEMIC PRESS INC., PUBLISHERS

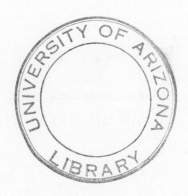

SECTION ON MICROBIOLOGY
THE NEW YORK ACADEMY OF MEDICINE

Officers
GREGORY SHWARTZMAN, *Chairman*
THOMAS P. MAGILL, *Secretary*

Organizing Committee for Symposium Number 8
E. RACKER, *Chairman*
G. K. HIRST
R. D. HOTCHKISS
A. M. PAPPENHEIMER, JR.

Preface

THE ORIGINAL PLAN of the symposium was to present a cross section of our knowledge of cellular metabolism in infected cells. In arranging this symposium it became apparent that the published data on this subject are few, scattered, and difficult to interpret. It might have been of some value to collect these data in a single volume and to assemble a pathology of infections at the metabolic level, but such an attempt seemed to be premature in view of the paucity of comparable data.

On the other hand important advances have been made in recent years in our knowledge of the metabolism and submicroscropic structure of animal tissues and microorganism. During the infectious process as well as in attempts at chemotherapeutic control, differences and similarities in the biochemistry of the host and the infectious agent assume a new significance. The concept of "unity in biochemistry" has for more than half a century oriented scientific thinking and experimentation in comparative biochemistry. The conspicuous lack of success of a rational approach to chemotherapy has served as a key witness for the "unitarians." However, the steadily growing recognition of the existence of alternate pathways, of qualitative and quantitative differences in enzymatic patterns, of differences in submicroscopic cell structure, permeability and rate of cell division have been quoted in favor of a "disunity in biochemistry." The assessment of those features that are not common to various cells might serve to provide us with a better understanding of the disease process as well as its control.

With these thoughts in mind the symposium was arranged and divided into two parts. One, on comparative biochemistry, dealing with differences in structural and metabolic patterns in hosts and parasites, the second dealing with metabolic aspects of the infectious process itself. The chapters in this volume represent the papers as they were presented at the symposium, though minor alterations in the sequence of presentation were made for the sake of continuity. In the first part some singular features of bacteria and helminths illustrating aspects of "disunity in biochemistry" were discussed by R. Y. Stanier and by E. Bueding, while the similarity of energy-yielding reactions was stressed by H. A. Krebs. The formation of adaptive enzymes has been studied for many years in microorganisms but was only recently firmly established in animal tissues; this subject was reviewed by

W. E. Knox. Some principles of a rational approach to chemotherapy were outlined by A. D. Welch.

The second part was devoted to a discussion of the infectious process. The peculiar environment of the host as a growth medium for bacteria was described by R. J. Dubos, while factors which contribute to bacterial diseases were analyzed by A. M. Pappenheimer, Jr.

Finally, aspects of virus infections were discussed. M. H. Adams reviewed the role of polysaccharides in the initiation of virus infections, and S. E. Luria summarized metabolic aspects of cytochemical and biosynthetic events in bacteria infected with phage. E. Racker dealt with alterations of cellular metabolism during some virus infections of animals and bacteria.

The discussions of the sessions were opened by the invited speakers B. Davis, S. S. Cohen and A. Lwoff. Their contributions as well as further discussions are included in this volume.

The invited speakers and discussants were selected not only on the basis of their outstanding contributions in the field of microbiology or biochemistry but also because it was expected that they would be free from fear of speculation and that they would follow the example of the turtle "who makes progress only when his neck is out."

E. RACKER

Yale University School of Medicine

Contents

x   CONTENTS

    *Present address The Public Health Research Institute of the City of New York, New
York, N. Y.

CONTENTS   xi

PART I

ASPECTS OF COMPARATIVE BIOCHEMISTRY

SOME SINGULAR FEATURES OF BACTERIA AS DYNAMIC SYSTEMS

BY R. Y. STANIER, *Department of Bacteriology, University of California, Berkeley 4, California*

Il faut avouer, dit Micromégas, que la nature est bien variée. Oui, dit le Saturnien, la nature est comme un parterre, dont les fleurs. . . . Ah, dit l'autre, laissez-là votre parterre. . . . Elle est, reprit le secrétaire, comme une assemblée de blondes et de brunes, dont les parures. . . . Et qu'ai-je afaire de vos brunes? dit l'autre. . . . Elle est donc comme une galerie de peintures, dont les traits. . . . Et non, dit le voyageur, encor une fois, la nature est comme la nature. Pourquoi lui chercher des comparaisons? Pour vous plaire, répondit le secrétaire. Je ne veux point qu'on me plaise, répondit le voyageur, je veux qu'on m'instruise.

VOLTAIRE, *Micromégas.*

I. INTRODUCTION

THE COMPARATIVE BIOCHEMIST is a scientist who seeks, as a rule, for the common biochemical principles which, his articles of faith tell him, are expressed in all forms of life. Certainly the search has been a rewarding one; and during the past 25 years the articles of faith so clearly enunciated by Kluyver (15) have proved an excellent guide for exploring the metabolic machinery of the living cell. Time and again it has turned out that biochemical information obtained from the study of microorganisms is highly relevant to an understanding of biochemical processes in vertebrates or green plants, and studies on these higher forms of life have in turn clarified microbial biochemistry. The history of the discovery of accessory growth factors and the elucidation of their metabolic function provide perhaps the most striking instance of this biochemical interplay, but other examples could be selected from almost any branch of biochemistry. Out of such successes, there has grown in some quarters a view which may be crudely expressed by the statement that the liver cell and *E. coli,* the meristematic plant cell and the purple bacterium, are sisters under the skin, their biochemical differences being principally ones of minor detail. However, a little reflection, which can be greatly stimulated by a judicious use of the microscope, suggests that there are, after all, some very marked differences between a liver cell and *E. coli;* and it seems not unreasonable to assume that the evident morphological distinctness of these two kinds of cell is the

3

outward and visible expression of less tangible chemical differences, more subtle than the gross catabolic differences with which biochemists have mainly concerned themselves in the past. Eventually, we must try to understand the *uniqueness* of the species and the group in biochemical terms, and such an understanding is certainly a prerequisite to the analysis of host-parasite relationships.

II. BIOLOGICAL ATTRIBUTES OF BACTERIA AND BLUE-GREEN ALGAE

From the time of Ferdinand Cohn in the mid-nineteenth century, many microbiologists have felt that the bacteria and blue-green algae together occupy a rather isolated position in the living word. It is difficult to explain the basis for this taxonomic hunch in terms of a compact definition; van Niel and the author (36) attempted to do so about 15 years ago, when the formation of a separate kingdom, the Monera, was proposed for these two microbial assemblages, but the formal differential characters which we thought up have not stood the test of time. The matter must, therefore, be put in a vague and general fashion: there is something about the cell structure of bacteria and blue-green algae which is different from the cell structure of other microbial groups—the remaining algae, fungi, and protozoa—and of higher plants and animals. For one thing, the cytoplasm in living cells of bacteria and blue-green algae has a very characteristic and unusual appearance, which in itself is well-nigh diagnostic. There is a total absence of vacuoles, and streaming movements are never detectable.

The singularity of the cell structure of bacteria and blue-green algae can also be documented with reference to a few specific cytological features. In eubacterial swimming forms the contractile locomotor organelle, although designated as a *flagellum,* is not structurally homologous with the organelles variously termed flagella and cilia in protists, plants, and animals. In these higher groups, contractile locomotor organelles are always composed of a bundle of longitudinal fibrils, characteristically 11 in number, of which two are structurally distinguishable from the rest (10, 11). The bacterial flagellum consists of a single very fine fibril without any evidence of internal structural differentiation (14, 39); Astbury (3) has described it as a "monomolecular hair."

In blue-green algae and purple bacteria, the photosynthetic pigments are not localized in typical chloroplasts, but are found in structurally much simpler bodies of submicroscopic dimensions (5, 32).

The question of nuclear structure in both these groups is at present very far from settled. Mitosis has never been observed in a blue-green alga, and as for the bacteria, the bulk of the evidence favors the view that the nuclear equivalents may not be strictly comparable in organization and mode of division to a typical nucleus in higher organisms.

One other biological feature may well prove after more extensive analysis to distinguish these two groups from other organisms: this is the mechanism of gene transfer. Considering all work on the three bacteria—pneumococci, *Escherichia coli,* and the *Salmonella* group— where the problem has been most extensively explored, one cannot help being struck by the fact that gene transfer on the bacterial level seems to involve the transfer of a limited number of determinants; either unit characters, or blocks of characters which could be construed (38) as being located on single chromosomes.

The question I propose to examine is whether there are any distinguishing biochemical features, either structural or dynamic, that can be correlated with the biological features that appear to set bacteria and blue-green algae apart from other organisms. In this analysis, I shall not be concerned with biochemical specializations that occur in small groups within the bacteria and blue-green algae—chemoautotrophy or nitrogen fixation, for example—since such properties are rare even within the assemblage as a whole. What we shall try to find are singular biochemical *group characters*.

III. OCCURRENCE AND ROLE OF DIAMINOPIMELIC ACID IN BACTERIA AND BLUE-GREEN ALGAE

1. *Discovery and Distribution*

A new amino acid, α,ε-diaminopimelic acid (DAP), was isolated by Elizabeth Work (46) from hydrolysates of *Corynebacterium diphtheriae*. Subsequent observations by Work and others (2, 4, 47) showed that it occurred also in the cells of other bacteria; but it has never been found in hydrolysates of plant or animal materials. Recently Work and Dewey (49) undertook an exhaustive survey of the distribution of DAP in microorganisms; their results, somewhat condensed, have been summarized in Table I. DAP is found universally in Gram-negative true bacteria, in photosynthetic bacteria, and in the one myxobacterium examined. In the Gram-positive group, its distribution is more spotty. The micrococci, the streptococci, and the mycelial actinomycetes do not contain it, but it occurs in rod-shaped lactic acid bacteria, propionic acid bacteria, corynebacteria, mycobacteria, and rod-shaped sporeformers, with the single exception of *Clostridium tetani*. Of the Gram-positive bacteria which lack DAP, the mycelial actinomycetes contain a new amino acid which is structurally related to DAP, being a methyl-substituted homolog (48). This compound is not present in the cocci, however. The fact that DAP is absent from the spherical and present in the rod-shaped lactic-acid bacteria is particularly remarkable since these two groups show far-reaching physiological, nutri-

TABLE I

DISTRIBUTION OF DIAMINOPIMELIC ACID IN MICROORGANISMS,
CONDENSED FROM DATA OF WORK AND DEWEY (49)[a]

	DAP Content
A. Unicellular Eubacteria	
α. Gram-negative groups	
1. Coliforms (8 spp., 20 cultures)	1 ++, 18 +, 1 tr.
2. Pasteurella, Brucella, Hemophilus (6 spp., 10 cults.)	tr. to ++
3. Pseudomonas, Vibrio (9 spp., 9 cults.)	1 ++, 7 +, 1 tr.
4. Neisseria (1 sp., 1 cult.)	+
5. Nonsulfur purple bacteria (4 spp., 6 cultures)	5 ++, 1 +
β. Gram-positive groups	
1. Streptococci, micrococci, sarcinae (7 spp., 8 cults.)	0
2. Rod-shaped lactic acid bacteria (1 sp., 1 culture)	++
3. Coryne- and propionibacteria (8 spp., 8 cultures)	++
4. Sporeforming rods (6 spp., 7 cultures)	2 ++, 3 +, 1 tr., 1 0
B. Actinomycetes	
1. Mycobacteria (4 spp., 4 cultures)	++
2. Mycelial actinomycetes (4 spp., 4 cultures)	0
C. Myxobacteria and Blue-green Algae	
1. Cytophagas (2 spp., 2 cultures)	+
2. Blue-green algae (3 genera, 3 spp., 3 cultures)	+
D. Other Algae	
6 species, representing 6 different phyla	0
E. Fungi	
19 species (Ascomycetes, Basidiomycetes, imperfects)	0
F. Protozoa	
1 flagellate, 1 ciliate	0

[a]On a dry-weight basis (whole cells) 0 = less than 0.02%, tr. = up to about 0.1%, + = 0.1–0.8%, and ++ = more than 0.8%.

tional, and biochemical similarities which have led bacterial taxonomists to place them in a single family despite their morphological differences.

DAP occurs in the three blue-green algae examined by Work and Dewey, but was not detected in representatives of six other algal phyla, in fungi belonging to the Ascomycetes, the Basidiomycetes, and the *Fungi Imperfecti,* in protozoa or in plant viruses. The presence of this amino acid is thus a sure indication of membership in the groups of bacteria and blue-green algae.

Studies on the intracellular distribution of DAP are still fragmentary, but the data of Work and Dewey show that in certain bacteria it occurs in bound form as a protein constituent. This is further supported by Salton's (26) observation that DAP is one of the amino-acid constituents in some bacterial cell walls.

2. Metabolic Role

There is evidence for a metabolic role for DAP, as well as a structural one, in some bacteria. Davis (6) has found that certain lysine-requiring auxotrophs of *Escherichia coli* which respond only to lysine excrete large amounts of DAP into the culture medium. This nutritional finding is neatly correlated with biochemical observations. Dewey and Work (8) found that the wild type of *E. coli* synthesizes constitutively a DAP decarboxylase which converts DAP to lysine, and that this enzyme is lacking in the lysine-requiring auxotrophs of Davis which accumulate DAP. The evidence for DAP as a metabolic precursor of lysine is, therefore, good, although not conclusive.[1] In nonbacterial systems, the biosynthesis of lysine has received little study; but it is known that certain lysine-requiring mutants of *Neurospora* can grow when supplied either with α-aminoadipic acid or with α-amino, ε-hydroxycaproic acid (12), neither of which can replace lysine for any of the lysine-requiring auxotrophs of *E. coli* examined by Davis (6). Furthermore, lysine-requiring *Neurospora* mutants cannot use DAP as a replacement (50). In summary, then, it seems likely that the presence of DAP as a protein constituent in most bacteria is correlated with the possession of a biosynthetic mechanism for the manufacture of lysine which involves DAP as a precursor, and which differs from the pathway for lysine synthesis in *Neurospora*.

A very interesting question now presents itself. Considering that DAP appears to have both a metabolic and a structural function in *E. coli,* is it possible that bacteria which lack DAP as a protein constituent nevertheless use it as a precursor for lysine synthesis, thus ranging themselves *biosynthetically* with DAP-containing forms? An indication that this may be so is provided by the observations of Dewey, Hoare, and Work (7), who found active DAP decarboxylases in two Gram-positive cocci, *Sarcina lutea* and *Micrococcus lysodeikticus*. Lysine-requiring auxotrophs of these two bacteria have not yet been produced, so that nutritional confirmation of the suggested biosynthetic role for DAP is lacking. It must also be mentioned that *Streptococcus fecalis* and *Leuconostoc mesenteroides,* which require lysine for growth and lack DAP as a protein constituent, cannot use DAP as a replacement for lysine (50). Of course, in the absence of

---

[1] See Adelberg (1) for a critical evaluation of the criteria used to assign precursor roles in biosynthesis.

positive evidence concerning the pathway for lysine synthesis by these two organisms, such findings do not necessarily disprove a general role of DAP as a bacterial lysine precursor. These lactic acid bacteria, belonging to a group whose very complex amino-acid requirements suggest a long evolutionary history of nutritional dependence, may well have lost most of the enzymes which control intermediate steps in the biosynthesis of amino acids.

The mechanism of lysine synthesis in mycelial actinomycetes, where a higher homolog replaces DAP as a protein constituent, has not been examined.

3. Concluding Remarks on DAP

Since some bacteria do not contain detectable amounts of DAP, this amino acid is clearly not essential for the construction of bacterial proteins *in general*. It would be of great interest to know whether, in bacteria where it does occur, DAP is incorporated only into molecular species of protein particular to these bacteria, or whether it also goes into proteins which are functionally and immunochemically like those of related, DAP-free bacteria. In other words, the DAP situation offers a perhaps unique opportunity to study the relationship between the amino-acid composition of proteins and their functional and immunochemical specificity. By far the best organisms for such a comparative study would be the two morphological groups of lactic acid bacteria, which together form a remarkably homogeneous assemblage in all major physiological respects but differ clearly with respect to the presence or absence of DAP.

IV. THE BACTERIAL CELL WALL

1. Chemical Composition

Eubacterial cells are always enclosed within a rigid cell wall which is distinct both from the inner cell membrane and from the outer slime envelope or capsular layer, although many bacteriologists differentiate in a very hazy fashion between these three structures.[1]

For many decades there has been speculation about the chemical nature of the bacterial cell wall, which can be found adequately misrepresented in

[1] One well-known bacterial cytologist recently stated (17): "On the basis of microchemical and macrochemical studies, the cell wall of *Acetobacter xylinum* appears to consist of cellulose." This bacterium undoubtedly synthesizes cellulose, and in large amounts; but cytologically speaking, the cellulose represents a capsular layer, comparable to the capsular polysaccharides of the pneumococcus in its extracellular location. For all that is known, the cell wall may be of an entirely different chemical nature.

almost any textbook of elementary bacteriology, but concrete information has only just begun to accumulate. Work on bacterial cell walls was involuntarily initiated by Weidel (43), who was attempting to isolate the receptor substances responsible for the adsorption of T-phages by *E. coli*. The receptors for T2, T4, and T6 proved to be attached to a sedimentable cell fraction, and Weidel was able to purify them considerably by allowing *E. coli* cells to autolyze, then treating the isolated cell debris with trypsin, to which the receptors are resistant. Preliminary analyses led to the characterization of this material as a lipoprotein of remarkable chemical and enzymatic stability. When at last the material was examined in the electron microscope, it was found to consist of nearly empty membranes, with shapes and dimensions similar to those of the whole cells. In other words, Weidel, a sort of bacteriological M. Jourdain, had spent many months isolating and purifying the cell walls of *E. coli* without knowing it.

About the same time, the isolation and purification of bacterial cell walls was taken up systematically by Salton and Horne (29, 30). They developed two procedures for this purpose. The more generally applicable is to disrupt a bacterial suspension mechanically in the Mickle tissue disintegrator or Raytheon sonic oscillator and then separate the walls from other cell fractions by a long series of differential centrifugations. The second method, applicable only to Gram-negative bacteria, is to squirt a thick cell suspension into hot water, which causes rupture of the wall and concomitant coagulation of the protoplast; after gentle shaking with glass beads, walls and protoplasts can be separated from one another by differential centrifugation. The identity of cell-wall fractions and, within limits, their freedom from contaminating cytoplasmic materials, was controlled by electron microscopy.

Some of the analytical data obtained by Salton (24, 26) with purified cell walls are given in Tables II, III, and IV. The most striking general finding is undoubtedly the great chemical complexity of the wall in all bacteria examined. Both amino acids and sugars are invariably present, and in the Gram-negative bacteria (unfortunately not a taxonomically well-distributed sample) lipids are also a major constituent. Nucleic acids were undetectable in all samples. The complexity of the bacterial cell wall seems to be far greater than the complexity of cell-wall structure in algae, fungi, and higher plants where the principal constituent is either cellulose (most algae and higher plants) or chitin (most fungi).

A second, no less striking fact which emerges from Salton's analyses is the great diversity of cell-wall composition in different kinds of bacteria. Walls of the two Gram-negative bacteria have an extremely high lipid content, whereas the lipid content of walls from Gram-positive bacteria is

TABLE II

SOME PROPERTIES OF THE CELL WALLS OF CERTAIN GRAM-POSITIVE
AND GRAM-NEGATIVE BACTERIA FROM DATA OF SALTON (26)

Organism		Mean determinations expressed as percentage dry-weight cell wall				
		Total N	Total P	Reducing substances[a]	Hexosamine[a]	Total lipid
Gram-positive:						
Strep. pyogenes		10.6	0.62	33.1	11.8	—
M. lysodeikticus		8.7	0.09	44.9	16.1	1.2
Sarcina lutea		7.6	0.22	46.5	16.3	1.1
B. subtilis		5.1	5.35	34.0	8.5	2.6
Gram-negative:						
E. coli	1.	10.1	1.52	16.0	3.0	20.8
E. coli	2.	10.0	1.52	—	—	22.6
Salmonella pullorum A.		6.4	0.88	46.0	4.8	19.0
Salmonella pullorum B.		5.5	—	—	—	—

[a]Determined after 2 N HCl. hydrolysis for 2 h at 100°C.
E. coli 1.   Preparation from 9 h culture of bacteria.
E. coli 2.   Preparation from 16 h culture of bacteria.
Salmonella pullorum A.   Cell walls prepared by mechanical disintegration.
Salmonella pullorum B.   Cell walls prepared by heat-treatment rupture.

low—so low, in fact, that it may reflect slight contamination with cytoplasmic materials. Notable also is the complexity of amino-acid composition in walls from Gram-negative bacteria,[2] and the rather simple amino-
acid make-up of walls from Gram-positive bacteria, *Streptococcus pyogenes*
excepted. This exception proved to have an interesting basis. *S. pyogenes* is
a group A streptococcus, characterized by possession of the M antigen,
which can be removed from intact cells by treatment with trypsin. Salton
could show by precipitin tests that the isolated walls still contained the M
antigen, and that it was removed by trypsin. Treatment with trypsin has no
apparent effect on the physical fabric of the walls, but abstracts their content of proline, arginine, cysteine, methionine, tyrosine, and phenylalanine.
As a result, the trypsin-treated walls fall more closely into line in amino-
acid composition with the walls from other Gram-positive bacteria, being

[2] Recently confirmed (28) for another, taxonomically quite distinct Gram-negative form, *Rhodospirillum rubrum*.

TABLE III

AMINO ACIDS AND AMINO SUGAR DETECTED IN HYDROLYSATES (6 N HCl. 24 h AT 100°C) OF BACTERIAL CELL WALLS FROM DATA OF SALTON (26)

Amino acid	Gram-positive					Gram-negative	
	Strep. pyogenes	Strep. faecalis	M. lyso- deikticus	Sarcina lutea	B. subtilis	E. coli	Salmonella pullorum
Alanine	+++	+++	+++	+++	+++	+++	+++
Aspartic acid	++	+	−	+	+	++	++
Glutamic acid	+++	++	++	+++	+++	+++	++
Serine	++	+	−	−	+	++	++
Glycine	++	+	++	++	+	++	++
Threonine	+	+	−	−	+	++	+
Lysine	++	++	+	++	+	++	+
Valine	++	+	−	−	+	++	++
Leucine/Isoleucine	+++	++	−	−	+	+++	++
Proline	+	−	−	−	−	+	+
Arginine	+	−	−	−	−	+	+
Cysteic acid	+	−	−	−	−	+	−
Cystine	−	−	−	−	−	−	−
Methionine sulphoxide	+	−	−	−	−	+	+
Methionine	−	−	−	−	−	+	+
Tyrosine	+	−	−	−	−	+	+
Phenylalanine	+	−	−	−	−	+	+
Diaminopimelic acid	−	−	−	−	+++	+	+
Amino sugar:							
Hexosamine	++	++	++	++	++	+	+

in fact qualitatively indistinguishable in this respect from *S. fecalis* walls.

The presence of rhamnose and hexosamine as the sole reducing substances in the walls of *S. Pyogenes* suggested that the group-specific polysaccharide, known to contain these sugars, might also be in the wall. Extracts of walls made by standard immunological procedures gave precipitates with group A antisera, thus confirming the inference (26).

2. Specific Enzymatic Destruction of the Cell-wall Fabric

Among the Gram-positive bacteria whose cell walls were analyzed by Salton were three species—*Sarcina lutea, Micrococcus lysodeikticus,* and *Bacillus subtilis*—which are killed by exposure to lysozyme. The walls of all three species contain the same sugars, glucose and hexosamine, and the walls of the two cocci also resemble each other in their remarkably

TABLE IV

IDENTIFICATION OF SUGARS IN 2 *N* SULFURIC-ACID HYDROLYSATES
OF CELL-WALL PREPARATIONS FROM DATA OF SALTON (26)[a]

Organism	Galactose	Glucose	Mannose	Rhamnose	Ribose
Gram-positive:					
Strep. pyogenes	–	–	–	++	–
Strep. faecalis	+	+	–	++	–
M. lysodeikticus	–	++	–	–	–
Sarcina lutea	–	++	–	–	–
B. subtilis	–	++	–	–	–
Gram-negative:					
E. coli	+	+	–	–	–
Salmonella pullorum A.	++	+	+	+	–
Salmonella pullorum B.	++	+	+	+	–

[a]*Salmonella pullorum* A.   Cell walls prepared by mechanical disintegration.
Salmonella pullorum B.   Cell walls prepared by heat-treatment rupture.

simple amino-acid composition. Hence it seemed possible that the substrate for lysozyme might lie in the cell wall, a hypothesis which was dramatically confirmed when Salton (25) found that isolated walls of *Micrococcus lysodeikticus* can be rapidly and completely dissolved by lysozyme. This observation was later repeated with walls from another sensitive bacterium, not included in the original survey, *Bacillus megaterium* (27). Apparently the linkages attacked by lysozyme are responsible for maintaining material continuity of the wall fabric, since the largest ultracentrifugally detectable fragments in lysates of *B. megaterium* walls have a molecular weight of approximately 20,000 (31). The chemical nature of the cleavage products has not been determined, but there is earlier evidence that the substrate for lysozyme is a mucopolysaccharide (9, 20). The walls of lysozyme-sensitive bacteria, which are chemically the simplest bacterial cell walls yet discovered, can thus be envisaged tentatively as consisting of a polysaccharide mesh made up of glucose and hexosamine units, within which are held, much like the pebbles in conglomerate, protein molecules of simple amino-acid composition and low molecular weight. In *Bacillus subtilis* the situation is probably a more complicated one, as evidenced by the increased number of amino-acid residues and the high phosphorus content of the walls.

A second enzyme with the ability to destroy the fabric of some bacterial cell walls has recently been studied by McCarty (18, 19). It is produced by *Streptomyces albus,* and can dissolve the walls of group A hemolytic streptococci. McCarty's experiments very strongly suggest, although they do not absolutely prove, that the group A polysaccharide of the wall is the actual substrate, so that the situation appears closely analogous to that just described for lysozyme.

Although other enzymes can selectively remove parts of certain walls (viz., removal of the M substance from *S. pyogenes* walls by trypsin), lysozyme and the *Actinomyces albus* enzyme are the only ones known to destroy structural integrity, and in each case their range of action is narrowly limited to a small number of bacteria which share common chemical features of cell-wall structure. Salton (28) has tried to isolate by enrichment techniques microorganisms capable of destroying purified walls of *E. coli* and *Rhodospirillum rubrum,* so far without success. For coliform bacteria, the observations of Weidel (44) suggest that certain of the T phages, notably T2, T4, and T6, may be good sources of cell-wall-destroying enzymes.

3. *Ultrastructure of the Bacterial Cell Wall*

In the cell walls originally studied by Salton and Horne (30), no details of fine structure could be ascertained by electron microscopy. Recently Houwink (13) has reported that the walls of two colorless spirilla show a very regular arrangement of spherical subunits about 120 Å in diameter; a similar ultrastructure has been observed in the walls of *Rhodospirillum rubrum* by Salton and Williams (31a), and may thus be characteristic of true bacteria belonging to this morphological group (Fig. 1).

4. *Analysis of Lysozyme Effects on the Whole Cell*

The finding that isolated cell walls of sensitive bacteria are rapidly lysed by lysozyme suggested that the killing of bacteria by this agent is a consequence of the enzymatic destruction of their walls. However, the well-known effects of lysozyme on sensitive bacteria are far more extensive than one would predict if this were its sole mode of action: as the name suggests, lysozyme rapidly reduces a suspension of intact cells to a viscous solution, or sometimes even to a gel, in which few formed elements remain. The apparent discrepancy led Weibull (41) to re-examine the effect of lysozyme on whole cells, using *Bacillus megaterium* as a test organism. It turned out that the lytic effect of lysozyme can be almost wholly prevented by conducting treatment of the cells in a solution of relatively high osmotic pressure, such as 0.2 *M* sucrose. Under these conditions there is a specific depolymerization of the cell wall with liberation of the enclosed protoplasts, which still retain the optical properties of whole cells, have flagella attached, and respire at an unimpaired rate. Suspensions of protoplasts remain stable for many hours if access of air is kept to a minimum, but apparently cannot grow in a medium suitable for

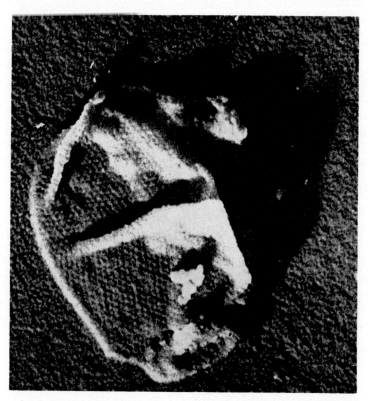

Fig. 1. A Cell Wall of *Rhodospirillum rubrum*, Showing the Hexagonal Pattern of Arrangement of Spherical Units, Each Approximately 120 Å in Diameter.
Compare with walls of *Bacillus megaterium* (Fig. 3), which show no regular ultrastructure. Electron micrograph by Professor R. Williams, of material prepared by Dr. M. R. J. Salton.

the growth of intact cells. Protoplasts can be immediately disintegrated by reducing the osmotic pressure of the environment (e.g., by sedimentation and resuspension in dilute phosphate buffer), giving rise to a highly viscous lysate like that resulting from lysozyme treatment of whole cells in a medium of low osmotic pressure. Thus the *direct* effect of lysozyme is indeed the specific destruction of the cell wall; but under the usual conditions of treatment this is closely followed by indirect osmotic lysis of the liberated protoplast. These experiments throw light on the function (or, perhaps better, one of the functions) of the bacterial cell wall; it is a corseting structure which prevents the rupture of cells existing in an aqueous environment whose osmotic pressure is low relative to that of the internal milieu.

5. *Immunochemical Implications*

Little advantage has so far been taken of Salton's isolation methods to study the relationships between the cell wall and the antigenic properties of the whole cell. His observations (26) coupled with those of McCarty (19) already show, however, that certain well-known antigenic components of streptococci are, in fact, either built into the physical fabric of the cell wall or intimately associated with it. The entire complement of bacterial "somatic" antigens may well be located in the cell wall, rather than in the cytoplasm proper. The chemical complexity of isolated cell walls is certainly sufficiently great to allow for the somatic antigenic complexity of such organisms as the *Enterobacteriaceae*. If this is a correct interpretation, the observed antigenic variation of individual bacterial species may reflect only variation in the chemical composition of the cell wall, or perhaps in the geometrical relationships of its component parts. The use of purified cell walls as antigens should permit a decision on this question. Furthermore, in species whose cell walls can be removed by enzymatic means, a whole new group of potential antigens—namely, those located on the surface of the protoplast—can be made accessible to more refined study.

The inference that somatic antigenic variation may reflect changes in the cell wall is made more plausible by Weidel's very pretty observations (43) on another type of specific variation in the properties of the cell wall. Walls prepared from a strain of *E. coli* B sensitive to phages T2, T4, and T6 can combine with all three phage types; but walls prepared from mutant bacterial strains resistant to one or another of these viruses can combine only with phage types to which the cells themselves were still sensitive.

IV. INTRACELLULAR LOCALIZATION OF ENZYMES IN BACTERIA

The last main question which I wish to consider is functional compartmentalization of the bacterial cell. Is it possible to discern in these organisms intracytoplasmic structures which, like the chloroplasts and mitochondria of higher organisms, are the unique centers for certain kinds of metabolic function?

1. *Localization of the Bacterial Photosynthetic Apparatus*

Even in the largest photosynthetic bacteria and blue-green algae, the pigment system of the cell as seen by light microscopy shows no evidence of localization, an observation which had long been construed as indicating that in these organisms chloroplasts are absent. Several years ago, Schachman, Pardee, and the author (32) undertook an ultracentrifugal analysis of the macromolecular components in bacterial extracts, and included in the survey one photosynthetic bacterium, *Rhodospirillum rubrum*. Much to our surprise, the entire chlorophyll-carotenoid complex in this bacterium was sedimented in the ultracentrifuge at an extremely high rate; in fact, it can be sedimented quite well without the aid of an ultracentrifuge, at gravitational fields of 15,000 to 20,000 g. The pigments of this organism are carried in particles of slightly variable size, whose diameter approximates 500 Å, and which have an average molecular weight (if that is the correct term) of around 30 million. Purified by differential centrifugation, these particles, which we designated as "chromatophores," show a sharp color boundary in the ultracentrifuge correlated with the only observable schlieren boundary. Indirect estimations, which are probably subject to a large error, give 5000 chromatophores as the number in each cell of light-grown *Rhodospirillum rubrum*. Thomas (37) independently observed these bodies in shadowed electron micrographs of crude extracts prepared from the same organism, as well as from purple sulfur and green bacteria. We have recently isolated chromatophores from a second species of non-sulfur purple bacterium, *Rhodopseudomonas spheroides;* their physical properties are very similar to those of the chromatophores from *Rhodospirillum rubrum,* and the entire chlorophyll-carotenoid complex of the cell is likewise located in them.

Studies on the localization of photosynthetic pigments in blue-green algae have been less detailed. Calvin and Lynch (5) found that the chlorophyll in extracts of *Synechococcus cedorum* could be sedimented at low gravitational fields, in association with particles slightly larger than the bacterial chromatophores; the phycocyanin remained in the supernatant solution.

Electron micrographs of isolated chromatophores (Fig. 2) show no evidence of internal structure, such as characterizes the plant chloroplast. In fact, chromatophores seem to be structurally equatable not with chloroplasts but with grana, and they have been so designated by Thomas (37) and Calvin and Lynch (5). This terminology is perhaps unfortunate, since the grana isolated from cells of higher plants are component parts of a larger structure, the chloroplast, whereas the chromatophores seem to be the structural units of photosynthetic activity in bacteria and blue-green algae. It is possible, of course, that chromatophores as isolated from bacterial extracts represent fragments of a larger structure existing within the intact cell; but if there were any significant degree of intracellular aggre-

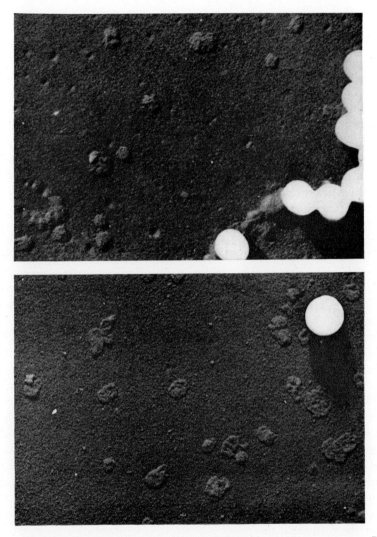

FIG. 2. PURIFIED CHROMATOPHORES FROM TWO SPECIES OF PHOTOSYNTHETIC BACTERIA. TOP: *Rhodospirillum rubrum*. BOTTOM: *Rhodopseudomonas spheroides*. The white spheres are polystyrene particles 0.25 μ in diameter. Electron micrographs by Professor R. Williams.

gation, a localized concentration of pigments within the cell should be observable by light microscopy, at least in the larger forms. On the basis of present evidence, it seems that the physical organization of the photosynthetic apparatus in bacteria and blue-green algae is different from that in other photosynthetic organisms.

2. Do Bacteria Possess Mitochondria?

Mudd *et al.* (22, 23) reported several years ago that a number of heterotrophic bacteria contain mitochondria. Their evidence for this was cytochemical, and rested principally on the observation that bacterial cells treated with the Nadi reagent, with Janus green, or with tetrazolium, show discrete stained granules. On the basis of their position, size, and number, these stained granules were also equated with the enigmatic electron-dense intracellular regions which have been observed in bacteria since the earliest days of electron microscopy, and which are occasionally misinterpreted (16) as bacterial nuclear structures.

Last year, when Weibull and Salton were working in Berkeley, we discussed the problem of these alleged bacterial mitochondria, and decided to attempt their physical isolation from extracts of bacterial cells which had been pretreated with a mitochondrial stain. Accordingly, Weibull turned his attention to this problem, using *Bacillus megaterium* as biological material and triphenyltetrazolium as a marker. The method used works admirably as a procedure for isolating the reduced product of tetrazolium, formazan, from bacterial extracts, but not as a means of isolating mitochondria. A careful re-examination by Weibull (40) of the staining of *Bacillus megaterium* with tetrazolium showed that the intracellular bodies which are colored in this treatment and which were interpreted by Mudd *et al.* as mitochondria are physical artifacts. If one watches the staining process continuously under oil immersion with phase contrast (which shows up the formazan granules very sharply), the formazan can be seen to appear first in the form of many barely resolvable granules scattered throughout the cell. These grow in size, then rapidly coalesce into one or two large granules, which clearly correspond to the structures described and figured by Mudd *et al.* (22) as mitochondria of *B. megaterium*. If cells in which such large granules have formed are disintegrated by sonic oscillation, and the resulting extract is then centrifuged to sediment the formazan, the practically colorless supernatant reduces freshly added tetrazolium almost as rapidly as the supernatant from a similarly prepared extract of untreated cells. We conclude, therefore, that the existence of mitochondria in bacteria remains unproved.

3. Evidence for an Intracellular Localization of the Bacterial Cytochrome System

The nature of bacterial cytochromes, long a subject of extreme confusion, is now being cleared up, largely by the studies of Smith, Chance, and their co-workers. The whole subject has been admirably reviewed by Smith (34). Aerobic and facultatively anaerobic bacteria display a variety of cytochromes, in many combinations; the complexity of the cytochrome pattern, when contrasted with the relative uniformity of cytochrome systems in other groups, insofar as they are known, recalls the complexity, earlier discussed, of cell-wall composition. Some Gram-positive bacteria (e.g., *Bacillus subtilis*) show a "difference spectrum"[1] whose peaks have a fair qualitative correspondence to those in yeast and heart-muscle preparations; but even extracts from these "typical" species are virtually devoid of cytochrome c oxidase activity, showing that their orthodox absorption spectra conceal functional differences from yeast or heart-muscle cytochromes. Other Gram-positive bacteria show obvious divergences from the typical cytochrome picture. The cytochromes of Gram-negative bacteria are even more singular, showing a uniform lack of α-bands corresponding to the typical bands of cytochromes $a + a_3$ and b. These α-bands are sometimes replaced by bands around 630 and 590 mμ (cytochromes a_2 and a_1, respectively) and at 560 mμ cytochrome b_1). In coliform bacteria an α-band corresponding in position to that of cytochrome c is missing; likewise in the *Acetobacter* group, where there is a new cytochrome with an α-peak close to that of typical cytochrome c. To quote from Smith (34): "Almost any possible assortment of the different cytochromes can be found in the group of bacteria examined, with the exception that cytochrome a does not occur together with cytochromes a_1 and a_2, and cytochrome a_2 does not occur in the absence of cytochrome a_1."

Recent studies on a number of different species (21, 35, 45) indicate that the cytochrome complement of heterotrophic bacteria is "particulate." This complex can be sedimented from extracts by high-speed centrifugation as a colored pellet; it can also be separated, though less cleanly, from the soluble proteins in extracts by precipitation with low concentrations (0.3 saturation) of ammonium sulfate. In one or two cases it has been shown that other enzymes are also exclusively associated with the cytochrome-containing particulate fraction; this is true in *Pseudomonas fluorescens* of the dehydrogenases for L-mandelic acid (35), glucose, and gluconic acid (45); and in *Acetobacter suboxydans* of the enzymes which oxidize

---

[1] The difference between steady-state oxidized and reduced spectra.

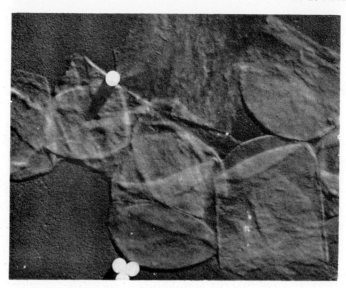

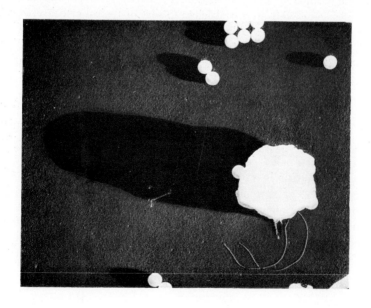

(*Opposite page, top*)

>FIG. 3. PURIFIED CELL WALLS OF *Bacillus megaterium*.
>
>Electron micrograph by Professor R. Williams, of material prepared by Dr. M. R. J. Salton.

(*Opposite page, bottom*)

>FIG. 4. A PROTOPLAST OF *Bacillus megaterium*, RESULTING FROM ACTION OF LYSOZYME ON CELLS SUSPENDED IN 0.2 *M* SUCROSE.
>
>Note the attached flagella, and also the density of the protoplast compared to ghosts (Fig. 5). Preparation and electron micrograph by Dr. Claes Weibull.

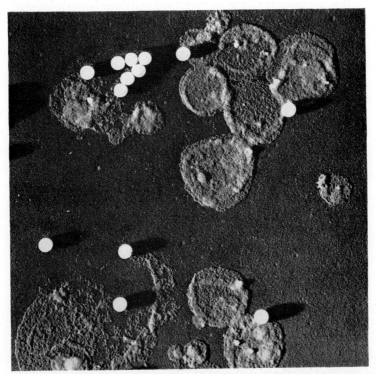

>FIG. 5. GHOSTS OF *Bacillus megaterium*, ISOLATED FROM AN OSMOTIC LYSATE OF PROTOPLASTS.
>
>One partially disintegrated ghost can be seen; the fine granules into which it is dispersed are of the same order of size as the "particulate fraction" found in extracts of bacteria prepared by mechanical disruption of the cells. Note the difference in fine structure between ghosts and isolated cell walls (Fig. 3). Figures 3, 4, and 5 are at the same magnification. The white spheres are polystyrene particles 0.25 μ in diameter. Preparation and electron micrograph by Dr. Claes Weibull.

alcohol, glucose, and lactate (34). Thus the particulate fractions appear to be enzymatically rather complex.

The physical properties of the particulate fraction vary with the method used for preparing the extract. As a rule, particles are more easily sedimentable from extracts prepared by alumina grinding than from those prepared by sonic oscillation, and prolonged sonic oscillation decreases the average particle size to the point where very high gravitational fields may be needed to bring about a complete sedimentation. It is improbable, however, that a true "soluble" preparation has yet been obtained. Centrifugal studies, and to a lesser extent electron-microscopic examination, have shown that the particle size in extracts prepared from bacteria by mechanical methods is always heterogeneous. It appears, therefore, that the bacterial cytochrome system and certain other associated enzymes form an insoluble complex within the cell, which becomes disrupted to a variable degree when the cell is broken by mechanical means. The morphology of the resulting particles is not suggestive of any particular native cellular structure.

Weibull (42) has made one very significant set of observations which may well provide the clue to the intracellular location of this insoluble enzymatic complex. When protoplasts of *Bacillus megaterium* prepared by controlled treatment with lysozyme in sucrose solution are washed free of lysozyme and then subjected to osmotic lysis, the largest formed elements in the lysate are empty vesicles (termed "ghosts" by Weibull) which are easily visible by high-power phase-contrast microscopy. They are of the same dimensions as the protoplasts, and evidently constitute a bounding membrane of some sort. Since lysozyme dissolves completely isolated cell walls (27), it is not probable that the ghosts represent a cell-wall residue; furthermore, they appear different in electron micrographs from typical isolated cell walls (compare Figs. 3 and 5). Weibull's interpretation, which seems the most reasonable one, is that the ghosts constitute bacterial cell membranes, perhaps in denatured form. They can be separated from the other components in osmotic lysates by differential centrifugation, and are estimated to comprise about 10 per cent of the bacterial dry weight. *Associated with this fraction is the complete cytochrome system of the cell*. It is, of course, possible that the cytochromes are merely occluded in or adsorbed on the ghosts, but one observation speaks rather strongly against this. The ghosts are very fragile, and easily break up into small particles of varying size, some of which, liberated from a disintegrating ghost, can be seen in Fig. 5. Brief sonic treatment is exceedingly effective in destroying the ghost structure. After this treatment, centrifugation at high gravitational fields sediments a pellet of uniform color, which shows that the cytochrome-carrying structures must be undergoing a fragmentation into particles whose average size corresponds closely to the average size of the ghost fragments, a situation compatible with the assumption that the cytochromes are built into the ghost fabric, but not likely if they are carried on a contaminating fraction. The sonic-treated ghost material is similar in its physical properties to the "particulate" fractions which have been obtained by mechanical disruption of many bacteria.

A great deal of further work on this problem is now needed, but I think Weibull's findings suggest that the bacterial cytochrome system, along with some other enzymes, may be a built-in part of the cell membrane, and not, as in higher organisms, a mitochondrial component (33). Such an interpretation would also fit with Weibull's observations on the course of tetrazolium reduction in cells of *B. megaterium,* which failed to reveal any well-defined intracellular localization of the primary sites at which formazan was deposited. To use a fanciful and not wholly accurate manner of expression, one could say that a very large part of the bacterial cell is perhaps the functional equivalent of the mitochondrion in higher organisms.

SUMMARY

Bacteria and blue-green algae are two groups with common biological properties which set them somewhat apart from other cellular organisms. An attempt has been made, with what success the reader can best judge, to bring together existing knowledge on the biochemical group characters which might also serve to mark these organisms as singular living systems.

REFERENCES

1. Adelberg, E. A. (1953). *Bacteriol. Revs.* 17, 253.
2. Asselineau, J., Choucroun, N., and Lederer, E. (1950). *Biochim. et Biophys. Acta* 5, 197.
3. Astbury, W. T. (1951). *Nature* 167, 880.
4. Bremner, J. M. (1950). *Biochem. J.* 47, 538.
5. Calvin, M. and Lynch, V. (1952). *Nature* 169, 455.
6. Davis, B. D. (1952). *Nature* 169, 534.
7. Dewey, D. L., Hoare, D. S., and Work, E. (1953). *Proc. 6th Intern. Congr. Microbiol.* (Roma) I, p. 79.
8. Dewey, D. L. and Work, E. (1952). *Nature* 169, 533.
9. Epstein, L. A. and Chain, E. (1940). *Brit. J. Exptl. Pathol.* 21, 339.
10. Fauré-Fremiet, E. (1953). *Ann. Rev. Microbiol.* 7, 1.
11. Gregg, G. W. and Hodge, A. J. (1949). *Australian J. Sci. Research Ser. B* 2, 271.
12. Houlahan, M. B. and Mitchell, H. K. (1948). *Proc. Natl. Acad. Sci.* 34, 465.
13. Houwink, A. L. (1953). *Biochim. et Biophys. Acta* 10, 360.
14. Houwink, A. L. and van Iterson, W. (1950). *Biochim. et Biophys. Acta* 5, 10.

15. Kluyver, A. J. (1931). The Chemical Activities of Microorganisms. University of London Press, London.
16. Knaysi, G. (1942). *J. Bacteriol.* 43, 365.
17. Knaysi, G. (1951). The Structure of the Bacterial Cell. Published in Bacterial Physiology, ed. by C. H. Werkman and P. W. Wilson. Academic Press, New York. P. 46.
18. McCarty, M. (1952). *J. Exptl. Med.* 96, 555.
19. McCarty, M. (1952). *J. Exptl. Med.* 96, 569.
20. Meyer, K. and Hahnel, E. (1946). *J. Biol. Chem.* 163, 723.
21. Moyed, H. S. and O'Kane, D. J. (1951). *Bacteriol. Proc.* 124.
22. Mudd, S., Brodie, A. F., Winterscheid, L. C., Hartman, P. E., Beutner, E. H., and McLean, R. A. (1951). *J. Bacteriol.* 62, 729.
23. Mudd, S., Winterscheid, L. C., DeLamater, E. D., and Henderson, H. J. (1951). *J. Bacteriol.* 62, 459.
24. Salton, M. R. J. (1952). *Biochim. et Biophys. Acta* 9, 334.
25. Salton, M. R. J. (1952). *Nature* 170, 746.
26. Salton, M. R. J. (1953). *Biochim. et Biophys. Acta* 10, 512.
27. Salton, M. R. J. (1953). *J. Gen. Microbiol.* 9, 512.
28. Salton, M. R. J. Personal communication.
29. Salton, M. R. J. and Horne, R. W. (1951). *Biochim. et Biophys. Acta* 7, 19.
30. Salton, M. R. J. and Horne, R. W. (1951). *Biochim. et Biophys. Acta* 7, 177.
31. Salton, M. R. J. and Schachman, H. K. Personal communication.
31a. Salton, M. R. J. and Williams, R. Personal communication.
32. Schachman, H. K., Pardee, A. B., and Stanier, R. Y. (1952). *Arch. Biochem. and Biophys.* 38, 245.
33. Schneider, W. C. and Hogeboom, G. H. (1950). *J. Natl. Cancer Inst.* 10, 969.
34. Smith, Lucile (1954). *Bacteriol. Revs.* 18, 106.
35. Stanier, R. Y., Gunsalus, I. C. and Gunsalus, C. F. (1953). *J. Bacteriol.* 66, 543.
36. Stanier, R. Y. and van Niel, C. B. (1941). *J. Bacteriol.* 42, 437.
37. Thomas, J. B. (1952). *Proc. Koninkl. Ned. Akad. Wetenschap. C* 55, 207.
38. Watson, J. D. and Hayes, W. (1953). *Proc. Natl. Acad. Sci.* 39, 416.
39. Weibull, C. (1948). *Biochim. et Biophys. Acta* 2, 351.
40. Weibull, C. (1953). *J. Bacteriol.* 66, 137.
41. Weibull, C. (1953). *J. Bacteriol.* 66, 688.
42. Weibull, C. (1953). *J. Bacteriol.* 66, 696.
43. Weidel, W. (1951). *Z. Naturforsch.* 6, 251.
44. Weidel, W. (1953). *Ann. inst. Pasteur* 84, 60.
45. Wood, W. A. and Schwerdt, R. F. (1953). *J. Biol. Chem.* 201, 501.
46. Work, E. (1950). *Biochim. et Biophys. Acta* 5, 204.
47. Work, E. (1951). *Biochem. J.* 49, 17.
48. Work, E. (1953). *J. Gen. Microbiol.* 9, *Proc.,* ii.
49. Work, E. and Dewey, D. L. (1953). *J. Gen. Microbiol.* 9, 394.
50. Wright, L. D. and Cresson, E. L. (1953). *Proc. Soc. Exptl. Biol. Med.* 82, 354.

SOME ASPECTS OF THE COMPARATIVE BIOCHEMISTRY OF *ASCARIS* AND OF SCHISTOSOMES*

By Ernest Bueding, *The Department of Pharmacology, School of Medicine, Western Reserve University, Cleveland, Ohio*

THE FIRST OBSERVATIONS on the metabolism of *Ascaris* were made by Weinland over 50 years ago (1). He reported that valeric and caproic acids are fermentation products of this parasite. However, the significance of these observations with regard to the metabolism of *Ascaris* has been questioned (2, 3, 4). It has been pointed out that in practically every other metazoa in which fermentation has been studied lactic acid has been identified as the product of anaerobic carbohydrate metabolism while the formation of large amounts of valeric acid by metazoa is most uncommon. On the other hand, the habitat of *Ascaris,* the host's intestinal tract, harbors a wide variety of bacteria, some of which are known to produce valeric and caproic acids (5, 6). Therefore, the occurrence of these acids in media in which ascarids had been incubated might be ascribed to the metabolic activities of bacteria. Also, the formation of these acids might be the result of combined biochemical reactions of helminths and bacteria.

It was felt that an answer to this controversial problem could be obtained by studying the metabolism of *Ascaris* in the complete absence of bacteria. This became possible by the use of a mixture of antibiotics which removed the bacteria from *Ascaris* without demonstrable injury to the worms. In fact, worms treated with antibiotics survived for considerably longer periods of time outside the host than did controls which had not been sterilized (7, 8).

Media in which bacteria-free worms had been incubated contained large amounts of volatile acids, while formation of lactic acid by these worms was insignificant. In 24 hr, 2.5 to 4 milliequivalents of volatile acids were produced by 100 gm (wet weight) of *Ascaris* (8). Over 40% of the steam-volatile acids had the solubility characteristics of volatile acids containing 5 carbon atoms, about 20 to 30% of them had those of C_6 acids, and 2 to 5% those of butyric and isobutyric acids. Of the remainder, 20 to

* The investigations of the author reviewed in this paper were carried out with the support of grants from the United States Office of Naval Research and from the Division of Research Grants and Fellowships, National Institutes of Health, United States Public Health Service.

biochemical reactions will be reviewed. The adult worm lives in the portal and mesenteric veins where the oxygen tension is relatively high (24, 25). Although the schistosomes take up oxygen their requirement for respiratory metabolism is low (26, 27). Survival and reproduction of the parasite depend almost entirely on the anaerobic utilization of carbohydrate (26, 28, 29). The rate of this utilization is extremely high. In 24 hr, the schistosomes metabolize an amount of glucose equal to their weight (26). In contrast to *Ascaris* schistosomes convert glucose quantitatively to lactic acid (26). In this respect the schistosomes resemble the tissues of the host. As in vertebrate tissues, lactic acid is formed via the Embden-Meyerhof scheme of phosphorylating glycolysis and the occurrence of enzymes involved in this series of reactions can be demonstrated in schistosomes (21, 30, 31). In view of this picture the question arose whether and in what manner the glycolytic enzymes of schistosomes are identical with or differ from those of the host. This problem was studied by the use of several glycolytic enzymes.

No significant differences were observed between the kinetics of the host's and those of the parasite's phosphohexose isomerase. This enzyme reversibly catalyzes the conversion of glucose-6-phosphate to fructose-6-phosphate. Almost identical pH optima, dissociation constants, and optimal substrate concentrations for both enzymes were observed. Furthermore, at equilibrium, the ratios between glucose-6-phosphate and fructose-6-phosphate were the same (21). These data suggested the possibility that the two enzymes might be identical. Evidence bearing on this question could be obtained by the use of an antibody against one of these enzymes because differences in their interaction with such antibodies would reveal differences in their nature. On the other hand, if the two enzymes were identical with each other they should exhibit similar behavior toward specific antibodies. Therefore, an attempt was made to obtain such an antibody by immunizing roosters against the isomerase of schistosomes. After repeated injections of this enzyme into roosters the sera of these animals markedly inhibited the activity of the worm enzyme (Table II). By contrast, these immune sera had no effect on the phosphohexose isomerase of rabbit muscle, indicating that in spite of the close kinetic similarities, the two enzymes are not identical. When the worm enzyme was incubated with the substrate before the antiserum was added a marked reduction in the inhibitory effect occurred (21). Therefore, it appears that antibody and substrate combine with the same site at the enzyme.

Another glycolytic enzyme of *Schistosoma mansoni* whose properties were studied was lactic dehydrogenase. Measurements of the rate of reduction of pyruvate to lactate revealed differences in the effect of pH on the activity of lactic dehydrogenase of rabbit muscle and that of schistosomes. The optimal activity of the worm enzyme was observed at pH 6.9 and that of the mammalian enzyme at pH 7.8. The optimal range for the oxidation of lactate to pyruvate was between pH 8.2 and 8.9 in the case of the schistosome enzyme and between pH 9.0 and 9.5 for the mammalian enzyme. Therefore, the pH optima for the schistosome enzyme were significantly lower in either direction of the reaction (31).

TABLE II

EFFECT OF IMMUNE SERA ON THE ACTIVITIES OF PHOSPHOHEXOSE ISOMERASE OF *Schistosoma mansoni* AND OF RABBIT MUSCLE

Immune serum against	Preincubation with	Schistosome enzyme, % inhibition	Rabbit-muscle enzyme, % inhibition
Control Serum	—	0	0
Phosphohexose Isomerase of Schistosomes	—	73	0
"	Fructose-6-phosphate	14	
Lactic dehydrogenase of schistosomes	—	0	

The optimal concentrations and dissociation constants for lactate were identical for both enzymes while those for pyruvate were 6 to 12 times higher for the worm enzyme. The corresponding figures for reduced or oxidized diphosphopyridine nucleotide were almost identical for both enzymes (31) (Table IV). These observations revealed some similarities, but also some marked differences in the kinetics of these two enzymes. Further evidence that the enzyme of the parasite differs from that of the host was obtained by immunizing roosters against lactic dehydrogenase of rabbit muscle. The sera of these animals inhibited the reduction of pyruvate as well as the oxidation of lactate, catalyzed by the rabbit enzyme (Table III). Control sera of untreated roosters produced no inhibitory effect. The immune sera against the rabbit enzyme significantly reduced the activity of rat-muscle lactic dehydrogenase, although to a lesser degree than that of the rabbit enzyme (32). Therefore, it would appear that the enzymes of these two mammalian species are similar to, but not identical

TABLE III

EFFECT OF AN IMMUNE SERUM AGAINST LACTIC DEHYDROGENASE OF
RABBIT MUSCLE ON THE ACTIVITIES OF MAMMALIAN AND OF
SCHISTOSOME LACTIC DEHYDROGENASES

		Lactic dehydrogenase of			
Substrates	Serum	Rabbit muscle, % inhib.	Rat muscle, % inhib.	Schistosoma mansoni, % inhib.	Schistosoma japonicum, % inhib.
Pyruvate +	Control	0	0	0	0
DPNH	Immune	68	39	0	0
Lactate +	Control	0	0	0	0
DPN	Immune	56	21	0	0

TABLE IV

KINETIC DATA FOR THE LACTIC DEHYDROGENASES OF RABBIT
MUSCLE AND OF *Schistosoma mansoni*

(*All values are expressed in terms of molar concentrations.*)

Reactions	Substrate	Rabbit enzyme		Worm enzyme	
		Optimal concentration	K_M	Optimal concentrations	K_M
Pyruvate → Lactate	DPNH$_2$	6×10^{-5}	1.5×10^{-5}	1×10^{-4}	2.5×10^{-5}
	Pyruvate	3×10^{-3}	2.5×10^{-4}	2×10^{-2}	3×10^{-3}
Lactate → Pyruvate	DPN	3.5×10^{-3}	5.6×10^{-4}	5×10^{-3}	6×10^{-4}
	L-(+)-Lactate	1×10^{-2}	2.0×10^{-2}	1×10^{-2}	2×10^{-2}

with, each other. Incubation of the immune serum with three other glycolytic enzymes of rabbit muscle resulted in no change in their activities (Table V). The enzymes tested were phosphohexose isomerase, aldolase, and phosphoglyceraldehyde dehydrogenase. Furthermore, incubation of crystalline phosphoglyceraldehyde dehydrogenase of rabbit muscle with the immune serum did not alter the inhibitory effect of the latter on mammalian lactic dehydrogenase (32). These observations demonstrated the specificity of the enzyme-antibody reaction. They indicated also that the antibody reacts with specific groupings common to lactic dehydrogenase of both rabbit and rat muscle. The immune serum against mammalian lactic dehydrogenase did not affect the activities of the lactic dehydrogenases of *Schistosoma mansoni* and *Schistosoma japonicum*. The possibility that this complete lack of an inhibitory effect was due to inactiva-

TABLE V

Effect of an Immune Serum against Lactic Dehydrogenase of Rabbit Muscle on the Activities of Glycolytic Enzymes of Rabbit Muscle

Enzyme	Per cent inhibition
Lactic dehydrogenase	43
Phosphohexose isomerase	0
Aldolase	0
Phosphoglyceraldehyde dehydrogenase	0
Lactic dehydrogenase (immune serum preincubated with crystalline phosphoglyceraldehyde dehydrogenase)	45

tion or destruction of the antibody by the extract of the parasite could be ruled out because the inhibitory effect of the immune serum on the rabbit enzyme was not altered by the presence of the lactic dehydrogenase preparation of the worms (32). Additional information about differences in the nature of the schistosome enzyme and of that of the host was supplied by the use of sera obtained by immunizing roosters against lactic dehydrogenase of *Schistosoma mansoni*. These sera markedly inhibited the activities of lactic dehydrogenase of *Schistosoma mansoni* and of *Schistosoma japonicum* but had no effect on the rabbit or rat-muscle enzymes (33). Pyruvate did not protect the enzyme from the inhibitory effects of the antibody. On the other hand, preincubation of the enzyme with reduced diphosphopyridine nucleotide markedly decreased the inhibition of the worm enzyme by its antibody (33). This protective effect suggests that the antibody interacts with the active center of the worm enzyme, possibly at the site where combination with reduced diphosphopyridine nucleotide occurs. It should be noted that the antiserum against the lactic dehydrogenase of the worms had no effect on the activity of phosphohexose isomerase of schistosomes and that, conversely, the antiserum against the isomerase did not inhibit the activity of the parasite's lactic dehydrogenase (21). This absence of a cross reaction supports the conclusion that the antibodies react with sites specific for a particular enzyme of the parasite rather than with groupings common to schistosome proteins.

Several differences between the properties of mammalian brain hexokinase and those of schistosomes were observed (30). The optimal concentrations and dissociation constants for adenosine triphosphate, magnesium, glucose, and fructose are considerably higher for the enzyme extract of the parasite. Another difference between brain hexokinase and the preparation from the schistosomes was revealed by the effect of glucose-6-phosphate on these enzymes. While this ester inhibits the phosphorylation of all three hexoses by brain hexokinase, it inhibits only glucose and mannose phosphorylation by the schistosome preparation. On the other hand, fructose phosphorylation is not affected. Similarly, sorbose-1-phosphate inhibits phosphorylation of glucose and of mannose, but not that of fructose. These results suggested the possibility of the presence in the worms of more than one hexokinase. This was indicated also by considerable variations in the ratios of the rates of phosphorylation of fructose to glucose, mannose to glucose, and fructose to mannose, by homogenates of different groups of worms. More conclusive evidence for the presence of several hexokinases in the worms was obtained by fractionation of schistosome homogenates with alumina gel Cγ: one fraction catalyzed the phosphorylation of glucose but not that of fructose or mannose, another contained fructokinase free of glucokinase and mannokinase activities, and a third one reacted only with mannose, but not with glucose or fructose (21).

Crystalline yeast hexokinase catalyzes the phosphorylation of glucose, as well as that of fructose, mannose, and glucosamine (34, 35, 36). The same is true for purified brain hexokinase (37). By contrast, in *Schistosoma mansoni* three different hexokinases are present, each of which reacts specifically with only glucose, fructose, or mannose.

In addition, schistosomes also contain another hexokinase which catalyzes the phosphorylation of glucosamine. None of the three hexokinases specific for either glucose, fructose, or mannose reacts with glucosamine while crude extracts of the worms possess glucosamine kinase activity (21).

It is concluded that differences in the enzymes catalyzing the same reactions in the parasite and in the host may occur at various levels. The phosphohexose isomerase of the worm could be distinguished from that of rabbit muscle only by the use of immunological procedures. They revealed the possibility that the functional integrity of the parasite's enzyme can be inhibited without affecting the enzyme of the host. The lactic dehydrogenases of schistosomes and of rabbit muscle can be distinguished from each other not only by their behavior toward specific antibodies, but also by their affinities for one of their substrates (pyruvate) and by the effect of the hydrogen ion concentration on their activities. In the case of the hexokinases of the host and of the parasite differences in the kinetics as well as in substrate specificities were observed.

The anaerobic and aerobic metabolism of *Ascaris*, as well as the nature of the glycolytic enzymes of schistosomes, demonstrate the existence of similarities as well as of differences in the biochemistry of the host and of the parasite. A great deal more work in this field is required until the information obtained from such studies can supply a new and rational basis for the chemotherapy of helminthiases.

REFERENCES

1. Weinland, E. (1901). *Z. Biol.* 42, 55; and (1904). 45, 113.
2. Fischer, A. (1924). *Biochem. Z.* 114, 224.
3. Slater, W. K. (1925). *Biochem. J.* 19, 604.
4. Slater, W. K. (1928). *Biol. Revs.* 3, 303.
5. Barker, H. A. and Haas, V. (1944). *J. Bacteriol.* 47, 301.
6. Bornstein, B. T. and Barker, H. A. (1948). *J. Biol. Chem.* 172, 659.
7. Epps, W., Weiner, M., and Bueding, E. (1950). *J. Infectious Diseases* 87, 149.
8. Bueding, E. and Yale, H. W. (1951). *J. Biol. Chem.* 193, 411.
9. Bueding, E. (1953). *J. Biol. Chem.* 202, 505.
10. Ciamician, G., Silber, P. (1896). *Ber. deut. chem. Ges.* 29, 1811.
11. Erdmann, E. (1902). *Ber. deut. chem. Ges.* 35, 1846.
12. Seidel, C. F., Schinz, H., and Muller, P. H. (1944). *Helv. Chim. Acta* 27, 663.
13. Neuberg, C. and Rosenberg, E. (1908). *Biochem. Z.* 7, 178.
14. Cram, D. J. and Tishler, M. (1948). *J. Am. Chem. Soc.* 70, 2438.
15. Fittig, R. (1894). *Ann. Chem. Justus Liebigs* 283, 47.
16. Power, F. B. and Rogerson, H. (1925). *J. Chem. Soc.* 101, 1, 398.
17. Seib, J. (1927) *Ber. Chem. Ges.* 60, 1390.
18. Von Brand, T. (1934). *Z. vergleich. Physiol.* 21, 220.
19. Von Brand, T. (1941). *Proc. Soc. Exptl. Biol. Med.* 46, 417.
20. Bueding, E. and Charms, B. (1952). *J. Biol. Chem.* 196, 615.
21. Bueding, E. Unpublished observations.
22. Laser, H. (1944). *Biochem. J.* 38, 334.
23. Chin, C. H. and Bueding, E. (1954). *Biochim. et Biophys. Acta.* 13, 331.
24. Blalock, A. and Mason, M. F. (1936). *Am. J. Physiol.* 117, 328.
25. Engel, F. L., Harrison, H. C., and Lang, C. N. H. (1944). *J. Exptl. Med.* 79, 9.
26. Bueding, E. (1950). *J. Gen. Physiol.* 33, 475.
27. Ross, O. A. and Bueding, E. (1950). *Proc. Soc. Exptl. Biol. Med.* 73, 179.
28. Bueding, E. and Peters, L. (1951). *J. Pharmacol. Exptl. Therap.* 101, 210.
29. Bueding, E., Peters, L., Koletsky, S., and Moore, D. (1953). *Brit. J. Pharmacol.* 8, 15.
30. Bueding, E. and Mac Kinnon, J. (1953). *Federation Proc.* 12, 184.
31. Mansour, T. E. and Bueding, E. (1953). *Brit. J. Pharmacol.* 8, 431.

32. Mansour, T. E., Bueding, E., and Stavitsky, (1954) A. B. *Brit. J. Pharmacol.* 9, 182.
33. Henion, W., Mansour, T. E., and Bueding, E. Unpublished observations.
34. Berger, L., Slein, M. W., Colowick, S. P., and Cori, C. F. (1946). *J. Gen. Physiol.* 29, 379.
35. Kunitz, M. and Mac Donald, M. (1946). *J. Gen. Physiol.* 29, 143.
36. Brown, D. H. (1951). *Biochim. et Biophys. Acta* 7, 487.
37. Crane, R. K. and Sols, A. (1953). *J. Biol. Chem.* 203, 273.

ENERGY PRODUCTION IN ANIMAL TISSUES AND IN MICROORGANISMS

By H. A. KREBS, *Medical Research Council Unit for Research in Cell Metabolism, Department of Biochemistry, University of Sheffield*

I. ENERGY-GIVING REACTIONS PROPER AND PREPARATORY REACTIONS

My starting point is the concept, now firmly established, that the free energy of the breakdown of foodstuffs, as a rule, is transformed into the "phosphate-bond energy" of adenosine triphosphate (ATP) before it can be utilized to do work, such as mechanical work in muscle or other structures causing movement, osmotic work in secreting glands or in 'active' transport, and chemical work resulting in syntheses.

I propose to consider and to compare in this survey some features of the mechanisms by which ATP is synthesized in the animal body and in microorganisms. The reactions which take part in energy production, in the light of the newer knowledge, may be divided into two groups. One comprises the reactions at which appreciable quantities of energy become available and are utilized for the synthesis of ATP. These are the energy-giving reactions proper. The other degradation reactions of foodstuffs all belong to the second class; they are all of a preparatory nature leading up to the energy-giving reactions proper. It is one of the unexpected discoveries in this field that the total number of energy-giving reactions proper—i.e., those which provide energy for the synthesis of ATP—is very small, considering the great variety of substances that can serve as ultimate sources of energy (12). In the higher animal only seven reactions—or correctly speaking seven types of reactions—are known where major parcels of energy are liberated and utilized and it is unlikely that an appreciable number of other reactions will be discovered. The seven reactions are listed in Table I. Two of these reactions occur in anaerobic glycolysis (all other steps of glycolysis being preparatory to these two steps). Three other energy-giving reactions proper occur when reduced pyridine nucleotide is oxidized by molecular oxygen through the electron-carrier chain, with flavoproteins and iron porphyrins as intermediates. A sixth reaction is the oxidative decarboxylation of α-ketonic acid and a seventh the oxidation of succinate (or cytochrome b) by cytochrome c. The mechanism of energy transfer is known for the two steps of anaerobic glycolysis and at

TABLE I

SEVEN ENERGY-GIVING REACTIONS PROPER

Two steps of glycolysis:

1. glyceraldehyde-P $\left.\right\}$ $\rightarrow$ $\left\{\right.$ 3-phosphoglycerate
   $+ \text{DPN} + \text{ADP} + \text{P}$ $+ \text{DPNH}_2 + \text{ATP}$

2. phospho-pyruvate $+ \text{ADP} \rightarrow$ Pyruvate $+ \text{ATP}$

Three steps of oxidative phosphorylation:

$$\text{DPNH}_2 + \tfrac{1}{2}\text{O}_2 + 3\,\text{ADP} + 3\,\text{P} \rightarrow \text{DPN} + \text{H}_2\text{O} + 3\,\text{ATP}$$

Oxidative decarboxylation of α-ketonic acids:

$$\text{R}\cdot\text{CO}\cdot\text{COOH} + \text{DPN} + \text{ADP} + \text{P} \rightarrow \text{R}\cdot\text{COOH} + \text{CO}_2 + \text{DPNH}_2 + \text{ATP}$$

Succinate $+$ ferricytochrome $\rightarrow$ fumarate $+$ ferrocytochrome
      $+ \text{ADP} + \text{P}$ $+ \text{ATP}$

least in principle for the oxidative decarboxylation of α-ketonic acids. It is still completely unknown for the remaining four reactions.

The utilization of the free energy of a chemical process requires a coupling mechanism specifically adjusted to the circumstances of the energy-yielding step. By reduction of the number of such steps to a minimum living matter reduces the requirements for specific enzymic mechanisms and thereby effects a striking economy.

The substrate changes taking place in the citric-acid cycle and in the reactions preparing substrates for entry into the cycle are thus preparatory to energy release, with the exception of the oxidation of α-ketoglutaric and other α-ketonic acids, and possibly the oxidation of succinic acid. This is due to the fact that the primary biological oxidizing agent is DPN or TPN, and with the exception of the case of α-ketonic acid no appreciable quantities of the energy appear in the oxidation of substrate molecules by DPN or TPN.

II. ENERGY-GIVING REACTIONS PROPER IN MICROORGANISMS

What I have said so far refers in the first instance to the tissues of higher animals.

There is no doubt that ATP also occupies a central position in the energy transformations of microorganisms. It is, however, remarkable that only in a few special cases, like that of yeasts, has the occurrence of ATP been established by direct determination or isolation. The occurrence of ATP in bacteria must be inferred from its actions in bacterial enzyme systems, for example in glycolysis.

There is also no doubt that the seven ATP synthesizing reactions found in the animal can also take place in a great variety of microorganisms, though not all species possess all seven reactions. The two reactions associated with anaerobic glycolysis may be taken to be present in all organisms which ferment glucose anaerobically, irrespective of whether the end product is lactic acid, or ethanol and carbon dioxide, or other substances containing between one and four carbon atoms like formic, acetic, butyric, propionic, or C_4-dicarboxylic acids, which may arise through glycolysis and secondary reactions beyond the stage of pyruvic acid. It is likewise very probable that the three reactions of oxidative phosphorylation occur in microorganisms. This is suggested by the presence in many bacteria of the required reactants—pyridine nucleotides, flavoproteins, and iron porphyrins—but direct evidence is still scanty. It is very probable that the two remaining energy-giving reactions proper (cf. Table I) also occur in many microorganisms but the actual extent of their distribution remains to be examined. It is uncertain, for example, whether the oxidation of succinic acid in yeast, which is very slow, is in this organism an energy-giving reaction proper, i.e., a reaction coupled with the synthesis of ATP.

In addition to the reactions found in animals there are other energy-giving reactions proper which occur in microorganisms only. One such reaction has recently been discovered independently by Knivett (8) and Slade and Slamp (18), and studied by Oginsky and Gehrig (15). It is the decomposition of citrulline to ornithine, ammonia, and CO_2:

$$
\begin{array}{ccc}
\text{NH}_2 & & \text{CO}_2 + \text{NH}_3 \\
| & & + \\
\text{CO} & & \text{NH}_2 \\
| & \xrightarrow{+ \text{H}_2\text{O}} & | \\
\text{NH} & & \text{CH}_2 \\
| & & | \\
\text{CH}_2 & & \text{R} \\
| & & \\
\text{R} & & \\
\text{(citrulline)} & & \text{(ornithine)}
\end{array}
\tag{1}
$$

This is a component reaction of the "arginine dihydrolase" reaction discovered by Hills (7):

$$
\begin{array}{ccc}
\text{NH}_2 & & 2\,\text{NH}_3 + \text{CO}_2 \\
| & & + \\
\text{C=NH} & & \text{NH}_2 \\
| & \xrightarrow{+ 2\text{H}_2\text{O}} & | \\
\text{NH} & & \text{CH}_2 \\
| & & | \\
\text{CH}_2 & & \text{R} \\
| & & \\
\text{R} & & \\
\text{(arginine)} & & \text{(ornithine)}
\end{array}
\tag{2}
$$

the first stage being the reaction

$$\text{arginine} + H_2O \rightarrow \text{citrulline}$$

Only recently (8, 18) has it been recognized that reaction (1) is an energy-giving process. It requires the presence of inorganic phosphate and ADP and the full chemical change is in fact:

citrulline | phosphate | ADP → ornithine + NH_3 + CO_2 + ATP

The reaction is in effect (and possibly, though not necessarily in mechanism) the reversal of a stage of the urea synthesis in the animal, and the arginine synthesis in living matter generally. It is estimated that reaction (1) yields approximately 11 kcal per mole, and this free energy is used for the synthesis of one pyrophosphate bond of ATP. The reaction has been studied in *Streptococcus faecalis* and also occurs in *Clostridium perfringens* (17). It is, no doubt, in part responsible for the accelerated growth of *S. faecalis* on a medium rich in arginine, arginine being a ready precursor of citrulline; but since arginine or citrulline are available only in very special circumstances, the scope of this energy-giving source is obviously limited. The idea is however of interest that this energy-giving reaction is probably an adaptation evolved from the reverse process which plays a part in the synthetic reactions of growing bacteria generally.

The mechanism of the ATP synthesis in this system is unknown. Oginsky and Gehrig (15) have suggested that a citrulline phosphate forms an intermediate but this is still a matter of speculation. Attempts to isolate such a phosphate have been unsuccessful.

It is commonly accepted that further anaerobic sources of energy are available to organisms which can effect oxidoreductions in addition to those of glycolysis. I refer to organisms producing, for example, acetate, butyrate, succinate, propionate, formate, hydrogen, butanol, acetone.

A mechanism by which ATP can be formed in these fermentations is presented by the following sequence (see 21 and 19):

$$
\left.\begin{array}{c}\text{pyruvate} \\ + \\ \text{coenzyme A}\end{array}\right\} \rightarrow \text{acetyl-coenzyme A} + \left\{\begin{array}{ll} 2\,H + CO_2 & (a) \\ \text{or} & \\ H_2 + CO_2 & (b) \\ \text{or} & \\ \text{formate} & (c)\end{array}\right. \qquad (3)
$$

$$
\begin{array}{c}\text{acetyl-coenzyme A} + \text{phosphate} \\ \text{(phospho-transacetylase)} \\ \rightleftharpoons \text{acetyl-phosphate} + \text{coenzyme A}\end{array} \qquad (4)
$$

$$
\begin{array}{c}\text{(aceto-phosphokinase)} \\ \text{acetyl-phosphate} + \text{ADP} \rightleftharpoons \text{acetate} + \text{ATP}\end{array} \qquad (5)
$$

Reactions (4) and (5) are absent from the animal and (3) only occurs in the form (*a*) provided that a hydrogen acceptor for the 2 H atoms is available, e.g., another pyruvate molecule. In the anaerobic lactic-acid fermentation pyruvate is quantitatively required as a hydrogen acceptor and unless alternative acceptors are available pyruvate cannot be dehydrogenated to the level of acetate. Alternative hydrogen acceptors are quantitatively unimportant in the animal under anaerobic conditions but many bacteria possess suitable acceptor reactions such as the reductive formation of succinate, propionate, butyrate, and butanol. It should be pointed out that not every acetyl coenzyme A molecule formed according to reaction (3) in bacteria can proceed to the stages (4) and (5). Some will be required for the formation of C_4 compounds via acetoacetate. There is no evidence showing that acetoacetyl coenzyme A formed as a primary product can react analogously to (4), but butyryl coenzyme A can react in Clostridia according to the following reaction scheme (19):

$$\text{butyryl Co A} + \text{acetate} \rightleftharpoons \text{acetyl Co A} + \text{butyrate} \quad (6)$$

The enzyme concerned, "coenzyme A transphorase," catalyzes generally the reversible transfer of coenzyme A from acetyl coenzyme A to other fatty acids. Reaction (6), in conjunction with (4) and (5), thus represents a mechanism of ATP synthesis.

The enzymes concerned with reaction (4), (5), and (6) can have two functions: anaerobically, proceeding from left to right, they yield ATP; in anaerobic organisms proceeding from right to left, they can convert acetic and other fatty acids into a reactive form.

The reactions here discussed may be the main source of ATP in propionic-acid bacteria or Clostridia growing anaerobically in a medium in which lactate is the main source of carbon, and also in Clostridia depending on the Stickland reaction as a source of energy.

The data on the free energy of formation of the reactants which have recently become available (4) make it possible to calculate the standard free-energy changes for a number—though not yet for all—fermentations. The results of such calculations are shown in Tables II and III. It should be stressed that the data must be regarded as approximate, mainly because they refer to standard concentrations, not to actual concentrations which are variable and therefore not definable.

To compare the different quantities of energy derived from glucose, the amounts obtained from one-half glucose equivalent have been calculated. It will be seen that substantially greater amounts of energy are, in fact, released in the more complex fermentations, enough, theoretically, to allow the synthesis of a second pyrophosphate bond for each half-glucose equivalent.

TABLE II

FREE-ENERGY CHANGES OF ANAEROBIC FERMENTATIONS[a]

Reaction	ΔG	ΔG per $\frac{1}{2}$ glucose eq.
Glucose → 2 lactate$^-$ + 2 H$^+$	−47.0	−23.5
Glucose → 2 ethanol + 2 CO$_2$	−55.9	−28.0
$1\frac{1}{2}$ Glucose → 2 propionate$^-$ + acetate$^-$ + 3 H$^+$ + CO$_2$ + H$_2$O	−113.2	−37.7
3 Lactate$^-$ → 2 propionate$^-$ + acetate$^-$ + CO$_2$ + H$_2$O	−42.6	−14.2
Glycerol → propionate$^-$ + H$^+$ + H$_2$O	−36.4	−36.4
Glycerol + CO$_2$ → succinate^{2-} + 2 H$^+$ + H$_2$O	−31.7	−31.7
Glucose → butyrate$^-$ + H$^+$ + 2 CO$_2$ + 2 H$_2$	−62.3	−31.2
Glucose → butyrate$^-$ + 3 H$^+$ + 2 HCOO$^-$	−61.4	−30.7
2 Glucose → butanol + acetone + 5 CO$_2$ + 4 H$_2$	−112.1	−28.0

[a]The data are calculated from those given by Burton and Krebs (4); ΔG at pH 7.0; standard activities.

Many microorganisms—the heterofermenters—can ferment the same substrate in several ways. Table III gives examples of heterofermentations in accordance with experimental findings by Harden (6), Scheffer (16), and Stokes (22) for *E. coli*. It is perhaps a little surprising that the energy yield of these complex fermentations is not appreciably greater than that of simpler forms of fermentations. This suggests that the significance of the secondary reactions in this organism may lie in the synthesis of intermediates required for growth, rather than in the supply of energy.

III. AEROBIC PREPARATORY REACTIONS IN MICROORGANISMS

The reactions of the tricarboxylic acid cycle are known to occur in many types of microorganisms but in some cases it is still uncertain whether these reactions play a major role in energy production. Rapidly growing microorganisms, unlike animal tissues, possess two types of rapid reactions. Apart from energy production, synthetic processes connected with growth take place and as far as the turnover of carbon is concerned both are of the same order of magnitude. In some microorganisms, e.g.,

TABLE III

FREE-ENERGY CHANGES OF ANAEROBIC HETEROFERMENTATIONS OF *E. coli*[a]

Author	Reaction		ΔG	ΔG (per $\frac{1}{2}$ glucose eq.)
Harden (1901)	2 Glucose + H_2O	→ { 2 lactate$^-$ + acetate$^-$ + ethanol + CO_2 + 2 H_2 + 3 H^+	−101.4	−25.3
Stokes (1901)	5 Glucose + 2 H_2O	→ { 2 succinate^{2-} + 4 acetate$^-$ + 4 ethanol + 6 fumarate^{2-} + 14 H^+	−288.7	−28.9
Scheffer (1928)	5 Glucose	→ { 2 succinate^{2-} + 2 acetate$^-$ + 2 ethanol + 2 CO_2 + 2 H_2 + 4 lactate$^-$ + 10 H^+	−276.4	−27.6

[a]The data are calculated from those given by Burton and Krebs (4); ΔG at pH 7.0; standard activities. The reaction schemes are formulated on the basis of the findings of the authors quoted.

Micrococcus lysodeicticus, Azotobacter or *Aerobacter aerogenes* grown in the presence of acetate, the evidence suggests that the cycle plays a major role in energy production, i.e., in the reduction of pyridine nucleotides. In many other organisms however, e.g., *E. coli* or yeast, acetate appears to be oxidized by a different pathway.

I cannot discuss the evidence in detail here (13). A few relevant observations are the following: *E. coli* fails to grow on media in which citrate is the sole source of carbon (10) yet if citrate is present in the medium together with glucose and a source of nitrogen, citrate is utilized (14). These observations may be interpreted as indicating that citrate cannot serve as a source of energy but may be used by growing cells for other purposes. Isotope data by Abelson *et al.* (1) also suggest that in *E. coli* the tricarboxylic-acid cycle supplies the carbon skeleton for a number of amino acids but is not the pathway of acetate or glucose oxidation.

Observations which argue against the participation of the tricarboxylic-acid cycle in the oxidation of acetate in yeast are the following: the oxidation of acetate in yeast cells made permeable to dicarboxylic acid by exposure to dry ice is not inhibited by malonate under conditions where the oxidation of succinate is inhibited; simultaneous oxidation experiments with C^{14}-labeled acetate and an unlabeled second substrate do not lead to the appearance of C^{14} in succinate, fumarate, malate, or α-ketoglutarate; the rates of oxidation of fumarate, malate, and citrate are very low compared with that of the oxidation of acetate. This all applies to conditions where the substrates are known to enter the cells and unless special intracellular permeability barriers are postulated which prevent access of the di- or tricarboxylic acids to essential sites within the cells, the conclusion must be drawn that acetate is oxidized through another pathway.

No positive statement can be made about the nature of alternative pathways in *E. coli* or yeast. Enzymes are present in these organisms which catalyze a direct oxidation of glucose via glucose-6-phosphate, 6-phosphogluconic acid, and ribulose-5-phosphate. It still remains to be shown that this pathway is connected with the energy-giving reactions proper leading to the synthesis of ATP. It is possible that this system is a mechanism for providing cells with reduced TPN for reductive syntheses. In any event, the direct oxidation of glucose does not touch the crux of the problem which is an alternative pathway of *acetate* oxidation. The suggestion has been made that acetate might be oxidized as coenzyme A derivative, glycolyl-, glyoxalyl-, oxalyl-, and formyl-coenzyme A being the intermediates. This is merely a tentative idea. In support it may be pointed out: (*a*) that no low molecular substances with one to six carbon atoms which might be intermediates in acetate oxidation have yet been found to undergo ready oxidation in yeast cells. This may be taken to indicate that acetate combines with a larger molecule before it is oxidized; (*b*) that enzymes which dehydrogenate the higher fatty-acid analogues of acetic acid (from butyric acid upward) in the form of their thiol esters have actually been demonstrated in animal tissues and in yeast cells.

A dicarboxylic-acid cycle of the type proposed by Thunberg (23) and by Knoop (9) has recently been discussed for molds and bacteria by Carson and Foster (5) and Ajl and Kamen (3) but Krampitz (11) has pointed out that the evidence is still to be regarded as inconclusive. On general grounds it may be argued that organisms like yeasts which can grow on acetate as the sole major carbon source are bound to produce a C^4-dicarboxylic acid before the reactions of the tricarboxylic-acid cycle can take place, and it seems feasible that the mechanism by which the C^4-dicarboxylic acid is formed might well have evolved in some species to one of the main energy-producing substrate reactions.

It has always been a striking fact that microorganisms are capable of deriving energy from a large variety of organic substances. Pseudomonads, for example, can utilize many organic substances that are inert in higher organisms. There is not much detailed information on the mechanism of energy production (i.e., ATP synthesis) from the substrates which Pseudomonads can oxidize, and on the question of the participation of the pyridine nucleotides. It would be interesting to examine whether the energy-giving reactions proper are the same as in most other organisms and whether the special feature of Pseudomonads and similar organisms is their ability to use a greater variety of organic substances for the reduction of pyridine nucleotides.

IV. ENERGY METABOLISM AND CHEMOTHERAPY

Before I conclude I wish to offer some comments on the question of whether differences in energy metabolism may form a basis for a rational chemotherapy aimed at interfering selectively with microbial energy production. In view of the similarities between the energy-producing mechanisms of host and infective agents the prospects of finding selective agents are not very good. Such quantitative differences between host and parasite that exist are not likely to be a basis for differential chemotherapy.

Energy production, of course, only represents one aspect of the metabolic activities of living cells; anabolic processes form another major part. Here again the pathways and mechanisms are generally the same in hosts and microorganisms, though there are differences in range: some substances may be synthesized only by the host or by the parasite. These qualitative differences may in some cases form a basis of chemotherapy, but what is perhaps more hopeful are the quantitative differences in the anabolic activities between host and parasite.

The rate of energy production may be, say, tenfold in the parasite, as compared to the host, and the growth rates of at least some organisms differ by a much higher factor from those of the host cells. Moreover, many bacteria (at body temperature) must grow or die and therefore a major slowing down of growth is more serious to the bacterium than to the host. Efforts to interfere with anabolic processes may therefore be expected to be more fruitful than efforts to interfere with energy production.

REFERENCES

1. Abelson, P. H., Bolton, E., Britten, R., Cowie, D. B., Roberts, R. B. (1953). *Proc. Natl. Acad. Sci. U.S.* 39, 1020; Roberts, R. B., Cowie, D. B., Britten, R. Bolton, E., and Abelson, P. H. (1953). *Proc. Natl. Acad. Sci. U.S.* 39, 1013.
2. Abelson, P. H. (1954). *J. Biol. Chem.* 206, 335.
3. Ajl, S. J. and Kamen, M. D. (1951). *J. Biol. Chem.* 189, 845.
4. Burton, K. and Krebs, H. A. (1953). *Biochem. J.* 54, 94.
5. Carson, S. F. and Foster, J. W. (1949). *Proc. Acad. Nat. Sci. Phila.* 35, 663.

6. Harden, A. (1901). *Trans. Chem. Soc.* 79, 610.
7. Hills, G. M. (1940). *Biochem. J.* 34, 1057.
8. Knivett, V. A. (1952). *Biochem. J.* 50, XXX.
9. Knoop, F. (1923). *Klin. Wochschr.* 2, 60.
10. Koser, S. A. (1923). *J. Bacteriol.* 8, 493.
11. Krampitz, L. O. (1952). *J. Cellular Comp. Physiol.* 41, *Suppl.* 1, 59.
12. Krebs, H. A. (1953). *Brit. Med. Bull.* 9, 97.
13. Krebs, H. A., Gurin, S., and Eggleston, L. V. (1952). *Biochem. J.* 51, 614.
14. Lominski, I., Conway, N. S., Harper, E. M. and Rennie, J. B. (1947). *Nature,* 160, 573.
15. Oginsky, E. L. and Gehrig, R. F. (1953). *J. Biol. Chem.* 204, 721.
16. Scheffer, M. A. (1928). Thesis, Delft: De suikervargisting door bacteriën der coli-groep.
17. Schmidt, G. C., Logan, M. A., and Tytell, A. A. (1952). *J. Biol. Chem.* 198, 771.
18. Slade, H. D. and Slamp, W. C. (1952). *J. Bacteriol.* 64, 455.
19. Stadtman, E. R. (1952). *J. Biol. Chem.* 196, 537.
20. Stadtman, E. R. (1953). *J. Biol. Chem.* 203, 501.
21. Stern, J. R., and Ochoa, S. (1951). *J. Biol. Chem.* 191, 161.
22. Stokes, J. L. (1949). *J. Bacteriol.* 57, 147.
23. Thunberg, T. (1920). *Skand. Arch. Physiol.* 40, 1.

METABOLIC ADAPTATION IN ANIMALS

By W. Eugene Knox*, *The Cancer Research Institute, New England Deaconess Hospital, Boston 15, Massachusetts.*

A STUDY OF the relation of metabolism to infection obviously must consider the biochemical reactions of both the animal host and the infective agent. In restricting this paper to a consideration of the former, I have in mind the importance of the host as the milieu for growth of the infective agent. Of particular interest are the differences between the metabolisms of the host and the infective agent, and the differences in the metabolism of the host from time to time. Probably many of the metabolic differences between the host and the infective agent which rational chemotherapy seeks to exploit are only quantitative. Kinetic factors will then determine the outcome of competitions for the same substrates. Chemotherapy must aim to affect favorably the competition between similar reactions as well as to block unique reactions of the disease agent. Kinetic factors, or at least changes in state, must also be considered in the concept emphasized by Dr. Dubos in this symposium: that a host *response* to the infective agent is a necessary condition of disease. The following is an attempt to rationalize the known metabolic plasticity of animals, as a necessary preliminary to any description of the role of the animal in his infection.

Analyses of enzyme levels show clearly that the complement of enzymes in an animal cell is not constant, but varies widely and quite rapidly. It is here assumed that the enzymes and the metabolic reactions they catalyze change in parallel. "Metabolic adaptation" will be used as the general term to describe this wide variety of changes in the metabolism of an individual. Metabolic adaptation in animals includes substrate-induced adaptations analogous to those familiar in microorganisms, and also hormone-induced adaptations which have been recognized only in animals. The adaptability of biological systems, long recognized as one of their cardinal features, is thus separated into two kinds: the adaptability of the species over many generations by genetic variations and selection, and the adaptability of the individual. Metabolic adaptation concerns only the latter type, and although it depends ultimately upon the genotype, it is determined during the individual's life much more by the aphoristic "nurture" than by "nature."

* This work was done under U.S. Atomic Energy Commission Contract AT(30-1)-901 with the New England Deaconess Hospital.

I. TRYPTOPHAN PEROXIDASE ACTIVITY—AN EXAMPLE OF METABOLIC ADAPTATION

Our interest in enzyme changes began with the observation that a rabbit given a dose of tryptophan in the morning could have up to ten times the normal activity of tryptophan peroxidase in his liver that afternoon. We had idly wondered, before that, how metabolic reactions were accelerated or slowed according to need, but until then we had never seriously considered that the metabolic machinery itself was labile in animals. The lability of the tryptophan peroxidase activity suggested that the rate of reactions in the cells might be governed by the changing amounts of the enzymes present. Starting with what we now know about the factors controlling the tryptophan peroxidase, I will explore this thesis: that the amounts, or concentrations, of enzymes in animal cells are continually changing, and that this is the basis of metabolic regulation and the basis of the physiological response of animals to changes in their external or internal environment. The particular role of this kind of response in infections remains quite unexplored at present, but its importance was noted above.

1. *Validity of the Activity as a Measure of Concentration Change*

When the activity of an enzyme alters, the primary concern is to decide if this is due to a change in the amount of enzyme, or simply to one of the many things which can change the activity of the same amount of enzyme in an assay system. The tryptophan peroxidase activity per gram of liver was much higher in those rabbits which had been given tryptophan some hours earlier (20). The same change was seen in rats, guinea pigs, and mice. This higher activity was found in assays using the liver slices, homogenates, or purified fractions of the livers of the treated animals. The assay conditions were those chosen after more than a year's study of the reaction mechanism of the enzyme. We were reasonably certain that the concentration of the enzyme was the only limiting factor. The elimination of inhibitors or increase in stability of the enzyme by the treatment of the animals was also excluded. By excluding known ways in which the same amount of enzyme could show more activity, it became most probable that the increased activity was due to an increased concentration of the enzyme formed in the liver by the treatment. With few exceptions, this is the only type of evidence available to show that the concentrations of the enzymes do actually change in metabolic adaptation in animals or in microorganisms. The term "concentration" is used with these reservations in mind, but the implications of an actual concentration change are important enough to support its occurrence with all available evidence.

a. Other Evidence of Concentration Changes. A recent experiment by Lee and Williams (24) provided additional support for the view that synthesis of new enzyme protein occurred. They found that the tryptophan-induced adaptation was blocked by the antimetabolite, ethionine. When sufficient methionine was also given to reverse the ethionine inhibition of protein synthesis, the tryptophan-induced adaptation of the tryptophan peroxidase occurred as usual. Tryptophan and the hormones which cause the change in enzyme activity when given to the living animal do not do so when added to cell-free systems of the tryptophan peroxidase (17, 19). This could also be interpreted as the need for protein synthesis, which does not occur in cell-free systems.

2. *The Rate of Adaptation and of Protein Synthesis*

The rate at which additional enzyme could be formed in the liver was determined by killing animals at intervals after treatment (Table I). In

TABLE I
TIME CURVE OF TRYPTOPHAN PEROXIDASE ADAPTATION

Hr after 2 mM L-histidine	No. rats	μM kynurenine/g wet liver/hr
0	22	1.2
2	2	2.3
4	2	8.4
5.2	1	11.8
7.8	2	10.4
12.5	2	1.9

5 to 7 hours after treatment, in this case with histidine, the enzyme level had increased manyfold over the normal level. Accepting the increase in activity as caused by an increased enzyme concentration, this means that new specific protein has been synthesized at a surprisingly rapid rate. But considering the great regenerative powers of the liver and the very small absolute amounts of protein responsible for this enzyme activity, such a rate of synthesis must be easily within the ability of the liver cells.

The important point so far as metabolic adaptation is concerned is that the response is specific and sufficiently rapid to be of physiological use to the animal. The response is an *adaptation* to the stimulus which caused the change.

3. *Two Separate Mechanisms of Adaptation*

The increase in the tryptophan peroxidase was obtained either by treatment of the animals with L-tryptophan, the specific substrate of the enzyme, or by the administration of certain other compounds which were not substrates. A substrate-induced adaptation like that known to occur in microorganisms offered a reasonable explanation for the first type of increase. But a second mechanism, perhaps hormonal, was suspected to account for the increase produced by the nonsubstrate compounds. Small amounts of epinephrine or histamine, or larger amounts of histidine or tyrosine, were effective (Table II).

TABLE II

SPECIFIC SUBSTRATE-INDUCED AND NONSUBSTRATE-INDUCED
(ADRENAL) ADAPTATION OF THE TRYPTOPHAN PEROXIDASE[a]

	No treatment	*0.25 mg Epinephrine*	*2 mM L-Histidine*	*1.5 mM DL-Tryptophan*
Normal:	9.3 ± 0.68 (6)	27.1 ± 2.21 (6)	39.2 ± 2.86 (8)	50.7 ± 10.8 (6)
Adrenal-ectinized:	5.6 ± 0.62 (5)	7.5 ± 1.68 (7)	9.6 ± 1.05 (6)	38.9 ± 7.97 (6)

[a]The activity (μMols of kynurenine per gram dry weight of liver per hour $\pm$ S.E.M.) was measured 4 hr after treatment of the adrenalectomized animals with tryptophan, and 6 hr after treatment in all other groups. The number of animals in each group is given in parentheses.

a. Substrate-induced Adaptation. Adrenalectomy abolished the effect of the nonsubstrate compounds, and only the specific tryptophan-induced adaptation remained (Table II). In specificity and other respects (17) the increase after tryptophan administration was comparable to the substrate-induced adaptations of microorganisms.

b. Hormone-induced Adaptation. The effective nonsubstrate compounds were, or could be, converted to pharmacologically active amines. These can release ACTH from the pituitary gland, and this suggested the mechanism for the second type of adaptation. Adrenalectomy abolished the response to the nonsubstrate compounds, which must therefore have acted by causing a hormonal secretion from the adrenal glands. The same effect showed the hormone-induced response to be different from the tryptophan response.

c. Cortisone-induced Adaptation of the Tryptophan Peroxidase. Cortisone has recently been identified as a product of the adrenal glands which can reproduce the increase in the tryptophan peroxidase caused by histidine or epinephrine administration, both in magnitude and in time of response (Table III) (19). The use of a different strain of rats was thought to account for the smaller changes in these experiments than in those of Table II. It is significant that adrenalectomy lowers the level of the enzyme, and that cortisone can raise it above the normal level in either

TABLE III

CORTISONE DUPLICATION OF THE CHANGE IN TRYPTOPHAN
PEROXIDASE CAUSED BY HISTIDINE[a]

	No treatment	Cortisone	Histidine	Cortisone plus Histidine
Intact Rats:	5.7 ± 0.34 (9)	14.3 ± 1.21 (9)	19.6 ± 1.33 (8)	18.3 (3)
Adrenal-ectomized Rats:	4.6 ± 0.36 (6)	12.7 ± 1.31 (6)	5.9 ± 0.64 (6)	18.7 ± 1.10 (6)

[a]Rats were given 1 mg of cortisone or 2 mM of L-histidine. The tryptophan peroxidase activity (μM kynurenine per gram dry weight per hour ± S.E.M.) was measured 5 hr later. Number of animals is given in parentheses.

intact or adrenalectomized animals, so that a wide range of control of enzyme concentration in both directions can be exerted by the adrenal glands. It is also important to point out that these effects of cortisone occur in 5 hours, after a single dose. Geschwind and Li (50) showed that ACTH can also increase the liver tryptophan peroxidase level under similar conditions.

4. Occurrence of Metabolic Adaptation under Physiological Conditions

The substrate-induced adaptation has helped to explain the derangement of tryptophan metabolism in pyridoxine deficiency (18). The activity of the liver kynureninase is not sufficiently decreased in pyridoxine deficiency to account by itself for the large excretion of tryptophan metabolites found in this condition after the administration of tryptophan. The kynureninase does not increase in concentration after tryptophan administration, so the adaptation of the tryptophan peroxidase which occurs heightens the disparity between the rates of tryptophan oxidation and of kynurenine removal. In this way the large amounts of metabolites, largely kynurenine and its precursors, accumulate and are excreted.

Increases in the tryptophan peroxidase level have also been observed in rats after 300 r X-irradiation, and after the stress of 12 hours without water. Cortisone release by these stresses, causing the hormone-induced adaptation, appears to be the most likely explanation for these changes. Alteration of the enzyme under these relatively mild conditions makes it more likely that changes can also occur with other exigencies of ordinary life, and more particularly with disease.

a. *Metabolic Adaptation during Tumor Growth.* Changes of the liver tryptophan peroxidase have recently been observed in my laboratory by Mr. Sumner Wood in mice bearing transplanted sarcoma T241. The changes in the enzyme level in this condition emphasize that the body as a whole responds metabolically to disease of a part; that this response may condition the course of the disease is a definite possibility. In the late stages of tumor growth, about 3 weeks after inoculation with tumor and shortly before the animals are killed by its growth and metastasis, the liver enzyme has risen to high levels, as shown in Table IV. An increased adrenal ac-

TABLE IV

LEVELS OF TRYPTOPHAN PEROXIDASE IN MICE BEARING SARCOMA T241[a]

| | Time after tumor inoculation | |
Controls	9–14 days	18–24 days
16.2 (28)	11.7 (24)	34.0 (9)

[a]The average activity (μMols of kynurenine per gram dry weight of liver per hour) was determined in animals at intervals after inoculation with the tumor, and simultaneously in the controls. Number of animals given in parentheses.

tivity arising from the stresses of advanced tumor growth would appear to be a reasonable explanation for this elevation of the enzyme concentration.

b. *Hormone-induced Adaptation with Lowering of the Enzyme.* The fall in the enzyme level during the second week of tumor growth and before the terminal rise (Table IV) was a most surprising finding. Its occurrence prompted us to look for an agent which might have such an effect. The usual approach might have been to look for an inhibitor of the tryptophan peroxidase, but we were concerned with finding examples of metabolic adaptation. Whatever may be the reason for the fall in liver tryptophan peroxidase during tumor growth, it led us to the effect of growth hormone. Growth hormone reduced the level of the tryptophan peroxidase to about half the normal value.

It is tempting to speculate that the biphasic curve of the tryptophan peroxidase levels during growth of a transplanted tumor represents the successive actions of growth hormone and of cortisone, released in turn as part of the body's response to the disease. However this may be, the level of the enzyme acts as an indicator, revealing changes in the physiological state of a tumor-bearing animal which were previously unsuspected. For the present purpose it is more important that a new hormone-induced adaptation was found, and one which demonstrated that hormones may decrease as well as increase the concentration of an enzyme.

II. A PICTURE OF METABOLIC ADAPTATION BASED ON THE
TRYPTOPHAN PEROXIDASE

The studies of this one enzyme, the tryptophan peroxidase of liver, lead to the conclusion that the activity, and probably the concentration, of enzymes in animal tissues *can* change. The changes can occur within hours, and are of sufficient magnitude to be of importance in the regulation of metabolism. Two mechanisms responsible for these changes have been identified. These are the specific substrate-induced and the hormone-induced adaptations. Particular hormones may act either to raise or to lower the enzyme concentration.

No consideration has been given here to the chemical mechanisms by which these changes might occur. The emphasis at present must be upon the physiological causes and consequences of metabolic adaptation. Those who would believe more readily that adaptations do occur, if they could see a mechanism by which changes could occur, can consult schemes advanced to explain enzyme adaptation in microorganisms (25, 30, 10). Advances in our knowledge of protein synthesis should be directly applicable to the chemical mechanisms involved in the sort of changes described here.

III. OTHER EXAMPLES OF METABOLIC ADAPTATIONS IN ANIMALS

The changes of one enzyme will not justify the theory that widespread changes occur in the metabolism of animals under physiological conditions as a result of alterations in the concentrations of many enzymes. There have been reported, from time to time, a number of instances in which abnormal enzyme activities in animal tissues have been found. A few of these changes, for the most part well documented, are given in the following Tables. They may well represent other examples of metabolic adaptation, involving different enzymes, but produced by mechanisms similar to those controlling the tryptophan peroxidase level. Other mechanisms besides substrate- and hormone-induced adaptations also appear to be operating under some of the conditions in which changes in enzymes have been observed.

It is unfortunate that negative instances—the failure of enzymes to change—have only rarely been published. Knowledge of these instances would enhance the specificity of those changes which have been observed. It is also regrettable that the enzymes most frequently studied are not those which would furnish the most information for the present purpose. These would be enzymes about which we have some knowledge of their physiological role. Instead, most determinations reported have been of enzymes like alkaline phosphatase, whose assay is simple but whose function remains a mystery.

1. *Examples of Substrate-induced Adaptation*

Some objections can be raised against most of the examples attributed to this mechanism. The clearest case, besides that of the tryptophan peroxidase, is the increase in the adenosine deaminase of the chick embryo (11). Injections of the substrate into the egg result in earlier detection of the enzyme and the presence of higher levels of it at hatching. Another example might be the liver arginase (26), which increases in concentration proportional to the dietary protein. The change could be due either to dietary arginine or to the total nitrogen, so far as is now known. The change could therefore be a more complex reaction than substrate-induction would imply. Whatever the mechanism, this case illustrates a type of information which can be gained from metabolic adaptations. The increase of one of the enzymes of the urea cycle under conditions of increased urea formation provides a unique kind of support for our belief that urea actually is formed by the reactions of the Krebs-Henseleit cycle (49).

2. *Hormone-induced Adaptation*

   a. *Thyroid-induced Changes of Enzymes (Table V).* The enzyme changes due to the action of the thyroid hormone given in Table V are often accompanied by the opposite effect with thyroidectomy or thiouracil treatment. The change in cytochrome C concentration is of particular interest, because this enzyme was determined spectrophotometrically. In this instance it is clear that the actual concentration, as well as the activity, changes.

The thyroid hormone does not produce a generalized increase in the concentration of all enzymes. A number are known not to be changed. The amine oxidase actually decreases, and in thyroidectomized animals it increases, and these changes affect the action of epinephrine in the animal (41). In the studies of the tryptophan peroxidase it was shown that a single enzyme could be increased by one hormone and decreased by another. Here it is seen that a single hormone can increase certain enzymes and decrease others. Further elaborations of the specificity of hormone actions will be found in other metabolic adaptations.

b. Metabolic Adaptation and the Mechanism of Hormone Action. The changes given in Table V concern enzymes acting in the terminal oxygen uptake as well as those acting upon substrates. The magnitude of the changes and time necessary for them to develop after thyroid therapy are of the same

TABLE V

SOME THYROID EFFECTS ON ENZYME ACTIVITIES
(Percent Change from Normal Levels)

Ref.			Thy-roxine	Thio-uracil	Thyroid-ectomy
(41)	Amine oxidase	Rabbit liver	−9	− − −	+15
		Rat liver	− − −	− − −	+24
(45, 6)	Cytochrome C[a]	Rat liver	+34	−16	−22
		Rat heart	+39	−26	−29
		Rat kidney	+22	−29	−28
		Rat skel. musc.	+21	−49	−47
(44)	Cytochrome oxidase	Rat liver	+46	− − −	− − −
(39)	Succinate oxidase[a]	Rat liver	+48	− − −	− − −
			+53	− − −	− − −
(39)	Hexokinase	Rat brain	0	− − −	− − −
		Rat skel. musc.	+66	− − −	− − −

[a]No effect with dinitrophenol.

order as for the changes in the basal metabolic rate in the whole animal. The enzyme changes could therefore be considered either the cause or the effect of the changes observed in the intact animal. It is particularly interesting that dinitrophenol, whose familiar action on oxidative phosphorylation also raises the oxygen consumption of the animal, does not change the concentrations of these enzymes. Since increased oxygen consumption by this mechanism does not require an increase in enzymes, it is unlikely that the increase with thyroxine is simply an adaptation to the higher oxygen consumption of that state. It would appear that thyroxine and dinitrophenol must bring about their similar effects in different ways. The simplest view would be that thyroxine increases the oxidative metabolism of the animal by increasing the concentrations of the enzymes concerned in these reactions.

The many failures to demonstrate the expected actions of the thyroid hormone on cell-free systems of appropriate enzymes would be explained by this interpretation. The hormone effects would be seen only in systems able to synthesize and change the concentration of the enzyme. Few cell-free systems can do this.

c. *Adrenal-induced Adaptations of Enzymes (Table VI).* The changes found after adrenalectomy and cortisone treatment may, when more ex-

TABLE VI

SOME ADRENAL EFFECTS ON ENZYME ACTIVITIES
(*Percent Change from Normal Levels*)

Ref.			Corti-sone	Adrenal-ectomy	Adrenal-ectomy +corti-sone
(9)	Arginase	Rat liver	+32	−69	−43
(8)		Rat kidney	−−−	−48	−−−
(1)	Catalase	Rat liver	−−−	−26	−−−
		Mouse liver	+11	−33	0
(46)	D-Amino acid oxidase	Rat liver	−22	−80	−21
		Rat kidney	0	0	0
(34)	Hexokinase	Rat brain (gray m.)	−−	+67	(0)
(47)	Proline oxidase	Rat liver	−−−	0	0
		Rat kidney	0	−60	0
(47)	Succinate oxidase	Rat {kidney, liver, and muscle}	0	0	0
(19)	Tryptophan peroxidase	Rat liver	+115	−31	+89

amples are collected, accord as well with our knowledge of the physiological alterations of the intact animal as do the changes found with thyroid treatment. The changes in activity of the enzymes concerned with degrading amino acids suggest such a parallel. Many enzymes are known not to change after adrenalectomy or with cortisone, so those changes shown are quite specific (47). The table also gives an example of another type of specificity of hormone action. Adrenalectomy decreases the D-amino acid oxidase in the liver, but not in the kidney. It decreases proline oxidase in the kidney, but not in the liver. The action of the hormone is directed toward particular enzymes, but this action is also determined by the tissue in which the enzyme resides. The complex of reactions occurring in each tissue must differ, and only by attributing a role to the environment could such an effect be explained. Besides the change of the same enzyme in one tissue while it remains unaffected in another tissue, examples are known in which the changes in a given tissue differ with the species.

The rate of occurrence of the enzyme changes which have been measured are in general somewhat slower than the changes of the tryptophan peroxidase. But another adrenal adaptation, due to epinephrine (and to the hyperglycemic factor) (43) is the change in the liver phosphorylase which occurs within minutes. This change probably does not represent a *de novo* synthesis of new enzyme, but nevertheless a change in the concentration of active enzyme, with more derived from a precursor.

3. Other Mechanisms Producing Metabolic Adaptation

a. Acidosis and Alkalosis. A particularly clear example of how metabolism is regulated by metabolic adaptations was furnished in the studies of Davies and Yudkin on ammonia formation in the kidney (5). Since the work of Van Slyke it was known that glutamine was the major source of urinary ammonia, and that it was formed by the action of glutaminase in the kidney. The remaining problem was one of regulation. If the substrate and the enzyme were always present, why was ammonia formed only in acidosis, and how was its formation normally suppressed? These studies showed that the glutaminase activity, and presumably its concentration, was nearly three times higher in the kidneys of chronically acidotic animals than in alkalotic animals, and about twice as high as in normal animals. The metabolic adaptations again provide a unique kind of support for the view that kidney glutaminase is actually concerned with ammonia formation. Proportionately great changes in the same directions were also found for the kidney glycine and L-amino acid oxidases. These enzymes would appear to be responsible for that fraction of ammonia not formed by glutaminase. The specificity of these changes was attested by the absence of any changes in the transaminases in the kidneys.

No alterations of substrate concentrations or of the hormonal state are known to account for the metabolic adaptations in acidosis. A new kind of mechanism, perhaps dependent upon the cellular concentration of certain metabolites such as ammonia itself, may well be involved in this situation.

b. Sex Differences in Enzyme Concentrations. The sex differences in activity of enzymes offer readily observable indications of the presence of metabolic adaptations, and many examples have been recorded. Many of the differences should properly be classified under hormone-induced adaptations, if the requisite studies have been made. This was done for liver catalase in mice, where it was shown that castration reduced the level in males to that characteristic of the females, and that testosterone administered to females raised their level to that of the male (1) (See Table VII).

TABLE VII

			Sex difference
Ref.			
(1)	Catalase	Mouse liver	♀ ½ of ♂
(38)	Cysteic acid de- carboxylase	Rat liver	♀ 70% of ♂
(13)	Pseudocholinesterase	Rat liver	♀ 3X ♂
			Diet
(13)	Pseudocholinesterase	Rat liver	−66% with 2 days starvation
(12)	Amylase	Dog pancreas	increased ⎰ high carbohydrate
(12)	Trypsin	Dog pancreas	decreased ⎱
(31)	Succinoxidase	Rat liver	−41% with high carbohydrate
			Age
(23)	D-Amino acid oxidase	Rat liver	increased to adult level at 21 days
(32)	Cytochrome oxidase	Rat liver	increased to adult level at 10 days
(29)	Alkaline phosphatase	Rat liver	+350% during liver regeneration

c. *Diet*. An additional characterization of metabolic adaptations follows from the fact that the response of the sexes to the same stimulus is different. The liver pseudo-cholinesterase of female rats, normally three times that in the male, drops much faster and proportionately farther with starvation than does the level of the same enzyme in males under the same conditions. This situation is reminiscent of the different responses of the same enzyme in different tissues, previously attributed to the different metabolic equilibria characteristic of each tissue, and of the differences in the adaptability to substrate of the tryptophan peroxidase in the liver of animals in different endocrine states (50).

d. *Age*. Differential developments of enzyme activities during growth of a tissue offer a fertile field for the study of metabolic adaptations, and clearly show that the functional activity of the tissue is closely related to its enzyme composition (27). The role played in tissue differentiation by the various mechanisms of metabolic adaptation presents a most challenging subject. Other changes, perhaps referrable to qualitative differences in the cell populations at different ages, have been reported (42).

e. *Drugs and Toxic Compounds.* Rapid alterations of enzyme activities after treatment with certain drugs, which in themselves do not affect the enzymes directly, are known to occur (Table VIII). These changes offer

TABLE VIII

CCl_4 Poisoning

Ref.			
(3)	Pseudocholinesterase	Rat liver	— 50% in both sexes
(35)	Conjugation of morphine	Rat liver	−66%
(35)	Choline oxidase	Rat liver	+50%
(16)	β-Glucuronidase	Rat liver	Severalfold increase

Colchicine Treatment

| (14) | Dopa decarboxylase | Rat liver | −60% } one day after |
| | Amine oxidase | Rat liver | no change } administration |

Altitude

| (21) | Carbonic anhydrase | Human erythrocytes | increased with residence above 4000 ft |

Seasons

| (48) | Cholinesterase | Guinea pig serum | low in summer (males only) |
| (2) | D-Amino acid oxidase | Sheep kidney | five times higher in fall than in spring |

to pharmacology a new hypothesis for the mechanism of drug action, to supplement the theory of actions by more or less specific types of enzyme inhibition. Alterations in the toxicity of certain compounds, as a result of metabolic adaptation, can also occur. The development of tolerance to drugs is a familiar but unproved example, possibly in some cases due to substrate-induced adaptation. The marked susceptibility of myxedemic patients to morphine and the decreased toxicity of acetonitrile for thyroid-fed mice (15) are other examples of drug action influenced by metabolic adaptations.

f. Seasonal Changes. Diet, light, temperature, and hormonal cycles are but a few of the variables that might be involved in the seasonal changes of enzyme activity which have been observed. The occurrence of seasonal changes does emphasize, however, the lability of the metabolic pattern of animals.

g. Disease. Table IX is appended for completeness. Its major effect must be to reveal how little we know about metabolic adaptations in disease as

TABLE IX

ENZYME CHANGES IN DISEASE

Ref.			
(37)	Aldolase	Rat serum	5- to 8-fold increase in tumor-bearing animals
		Rat liver	lowered in tumor-bearing animals
(22)	Carbonic anhydrase	Human	
(4)		erythrocytes	lowered in pneumonia, tuberculosis
(36)	Histaminase	Rabbit serum	+126% in anaphylaxis
(7)		Rabbit kidney	no change in anaphylaxis
(40)	Lipase	Rabbit serum	+27% after typhoid vaccine
(28)		Rabbit serum	increased in experimental peritonitis
(28)	Amylase	Rabbit serum	no change in experimental peritonitis
(33)	Fibrinolysin	Human plasma	increased 4-fold after pneumonia

yet. It is in this field, in the action and reaction of disease and host, that a knowledge of the basic metabolic adaptation mechanisms could most profitably be used.

SUMMARY

A number of instances have been considered in which enzyme concentrations in animal cells appear to change. This general phenomenon, called metabolic adaptation, occurs widely in different species and tissues and involves a large variety of enzymes. The changes recorded are often large and rapid enough to be of importance in regulating metabolism. Although the fundamental reactions permitting changes in cellular enzyme concentrations are unknown, at least two different mechanisms leading to such changes have been distinguished. These are substrate-induced and hormone-induced adaptations. Some factors determining the specificity of hormone action were cited. The physiological appropriateness of these changes is obvious, as in the increase of tryptophan peroxidase by tryptophan administration, the increase of oxidative enzymes by thyroxine, and the increase of ammonia-forming enzymes in the kidney by acidosis. Instances of metabolic adaptations in diverse physiological states, including disease, have been noted. More detailed knowledge of the various metabolic adaptations which can occur would simplify our analysis of the host response to disease. This knowledge would also give us a dynamic picture in biochemical terms of the organism as it responds to the action of hormones, drugs, and environmental conditions.

REFERENCES

1. Adams, D. H. (1952). *Biochem. J.* 50, 486.
2. Bender, A. E., and Krebs, H. A. (1950). *Biochem. J.* 46, 210.
3. Brown, L. M., and Harrison, M. F. (1951). *Nature* 168, 83.
4. Cattaneo, C., and Bassani, B. (1946). *Ann. 1st. "Carlo Forlanini"* 9, 9.
5. Davies, B. M. A., and Yudkin, J. (1952). *Biochem. J.* 52, 407.
6. Drabkin, D. L. (1950). *J. Biol. Chem.* 182, 335.
7. Eisen, H. (1946). *Am. J. Physiol.* 146, 56.
8. Folley, S. J., and Greenbaum, A. L. (1948). *Biochem. J.* 43, 581.
9. Fraenkel-Conrat, H., Simpson, M. E., and Evans, H. M. (1943). *J. Biol. Chem.* 147, 99.
10. Gale, E. F. (1943). *Bacteriol. Revs.* 7, 139.
11. Gordon, M. W. (1952). *Federation Proc.* 11, 220.
12. Grossman, M. I., Greengaard, H., and Ivy, A. C. (1942-3). *Am. J. Physiol.* 138, 467.
13. Harrison, M. F., and Brown, L. M. (1951). *Biochem. J.* 48, 151.
14. Hawkins, J., and Walker, J. M. (1952). *Brit. J. Pharmacol.* 7, 152.
15. Hunt, R. (1923). *Am. J. Physiol.* 63, 257.
16. Kerr, L. M. H., Campbell, J. E., and Levvy, E. A. (1949). *Biochem. J.* 34, 488.
17. Knox, W. E. (1951). *Brit. J. Exptl. Pathol.* 32, 462.
18. Knox, W. E. (1953). *Biochem. J.* 53, 379.
19. Knox, W. E., and Auerbach, V. H. Unpublished observations.
20. Knox, W. E., and Mehler, A. H. (1951). *Science* 113, 237.
21. Kreps, E. M. (1945). *Bull. acad. sci. URSS Sér. biol.* 197.
22. Kreps, E. M., and Chenykov, E. (1945). *Khirurgiya* 15, 22.
23. Kuniati, K., and Kensler, C. J. (1952). *Federation Proc.* 11, 365.
24. Lee, N. D., and Williams, R. H. (1952). *Biochim. et Biophys. Acta* 9, 698.
25. Mandelstam, J. (1952). *Biochem. J.* 51, 674.
26. Mandelstam, J., and Yudkin, J. (1952). *Biochem. J.* 51, 681.
27. Moog, F. (1952). *Ann. N. Y. Acad. Sci.* 55, Art. 2, 57.
28. Nemir, J., Hawthorne, H. R., and Lecrone, B. L. (1949). *Arch. Surg.* 59, 337.
29. Oppenheimer, M. J., and Flack, E. V. (1947). *Am. J. Physiol.* 149, 418.
30. Pollock, M. R. (1953). *Brit. J. Exptl. Pathol.* 34, 251.
31. Potter, V. R., and King, H. L. (1947). *Arch. Biochem.* 12, 241.
32. Potter, V. R., Schneider, W. C., and Liebl, G. J. (1945). *Cancer Research* 5, 21.
33. Ratnoff, O. D. (1951). *Bull. Johns Hopkins Hosp.* 88, 304.

34. Reiss, M., and Rees, D. S. (1947). *Endocrinology* 41, 437.
35. Richter, M. L. (1951). *J. Pharmacol. Exptl. Therap.* 102, 94.
36. Rose, B., and Leger, J. (1952). *Proc. Soc. Exptl. Biol. Med.* 79, 379.
37. Sibley, J. A., and Lehninger, A. L. (1949). *J. Natl. Cancer Inst.* 9, 303.
38. Sloan-Stanley, G. H. (1949). *Biochem. J.* 45, 556.
39. Smith, R. H., and Williams-Ashman, H. G. (1951). *Biochim. et Biophys. Acta* 7, 295.
40. Solarino, G., and Tripodo, C. (1948). *Boll. 1st. sieroterap. milan.* 27, 161.
41. Spinks, A., and Burn, J. H. (1952). *Brit. J. Pharmacol.* 7, 93.
42. Stern, K., Birmingham, M. K., Cullen, A., and Richer, R. (1951). *J. Clin. Invest.* 30, 84.
43. Sutherland, E. W. (1952). Phosphorus Metabolism, ed. by W. D. McElroy and B. Glass, p. 577. The Johns Hopkins Press, Baltimore.
44. Tipton, S. R., Leath, M. J., Tipton, I. H., and Nixon, W. L. (1945). *Am. J. Physiol.* 145, 693.
45. Tissieres, A. (1946). *Arch. intern. physiol.* 54, 305.
46. Umbreit, W. W., and Tonhazy, N. E. (1951). *Arch. Biochem. and Biophys.* 32, 96.
47. Umbreit, W. W., and Tonhazy, N. E. (1951). *J. Biol. Chem.* 191, 249.
48. van Wattenwyl, H., Bissegger, A., Maietz, A., and Zeller, E. A. (1943). *Helv. Chim. Acta.* 26, 2063.
49. Yudkin, J. (1952). L. Farkes Memorial Volume, Research Council of Israel, Jerusalem.
50. Geschwind, I. I., and Li, C. H. (1953). *Nature* 172, 732.

METABOLIC APPROACHES TO CHEMOTHERAPY

By Arnold D. Welch, *Department of Pharmacology, Yale University, School of Medicine, New Haven, Connecticut*

I. INTRODUCTION

It is the purpose of this article not only to place renewed emphasis on the important contributions which have been made and can be anticipated from metabolic approaches to chemotherapy, but also to call attention to the fallacious foundation for certain mild polemics of the recent past. These controversies may perhaps be attributed largely to two somewhat over-emphasized viewpoints: one is the interpretation, by the so-called empiricists, that those who stress the biochemical approach sometimes appear to claim a monopoly on intelligence, while the other is the implication that the metabolic approach is pure, wholly rational, and unsullied by the taint of empiricism.

Careful scrutiny of the important advances which have been made in chemotherapy during the past half-century will show that nearly all have been based primarily on empirical observations. On the other hand, none of the most empirical of these advances has been so dependent on chance that the contributions of the human mind should be cynically minimized. To an increasing degree the chemotherapeutic "empiricist" is being forced to become a "metabolist," while the latter often finds that metabolic leads are in themselves no magic "Sesame" to the design of unique chemotherapeutic agents.

In a brief article of this nature no attempt could be made to cover the field comprehensively. The selections made should be regarded as reflections of the interests of the reviewer and not in any sense as an implied criticism of work which has not been discussed in this paper.

II. DEVELOPMENT OF AN ANTAGONIST OF ARSENICAL TOXICITY ON THE BASIS OF METABOLIC FINDINGS

In a discussion of recent metabolic approaches to chemotherapy it is particularly pertinent to begin with the studies of Peters, Stocken, and Thompson (50) at Oxford which led to the development of the antagonist dimercaprol (BAL). Although it may be asked whether this is a chemotherapeutic agent, since the term chemotherapy is usually restricted to the treatment of infections with parasitic organisms, the reasons for such a limitation are not altogether compelling. Actually a more general application of the term chemotherapy is indicated by its now common use in connection with the study of chemical agents which exhibit inhibitory effects on the development of certain types of neoplasms. Accordingly,

61

from a broader point of view, and for the purposes of our discussion, the development of a potent means of combatting the poisonous effects of arsenical compounds may be regarded as a form of chemotherapeutic research. Certainly, this development afforded an outstanding example of the contribution of metabolic reasoning to the partial solution, through the design of an effective antagonist, of a very serious problem of toxicology.

Voegtlin and his colleagues had demonstrated in 1923 (60) that the toxic and trypanocidal activities of certain benzene-substituted arsenicals could be nullified by glutathione, and had proposed that these agents exert their effects by reacting with glutathione [or other sulfhydryl-containing compounds] in tissues and in parasites. According to this view, the sulfhydryl (SH) group could be regarded as the chemo-receptor for arsenic, which had been suggested by Ehrlich, but proof of this attractive hypothesis, of course, was not available.

When, at the outbreak of World War II, belated recognition was given to the serious problems created by the existence of chlorovinyl-dichloroarsine (Lewisite) and other arsenical "war gases," the desperate need for a means of counteracting the effects of these agents was appreciated. Accepting as a working hypothesis the deductions derived from earlier studies, the Oxford investigators tested many monothiols, but among these found no compound with promising activity as a "detoxifying agent." When studies were made, however, of the reactions between Lewisite and the thiol protein, kerateine, Stocken and Thompson (59) conceived the idea that such compounds of arsenic exert their toxicity by combining with two thiol groups closely situated in space, forming thereby a comparatively stable ring.

$$R-As \underset{S-C}{\overset{S-C}{\Big\langle}} \ \ \text{Protein residue}$$

This concept led at once to the synthesis of compounds containing two thiol groups on adjacent carbon atoms, and these formed with arsenicals even more stable five-membered ring compounds. The least toxic of the substances made was a dimercaptopropanol, CH_2-(SH)-CH(SH)-CH_2OH, long referred to as British Anti-Lewisite or BAL, and now named Dimercaprol. In addition to work with kerateine, metabolic studies of the action *in vitro* of arsenicals and various thiols, especially BAL, on another "model" system, the thiol-dependent pyruvate oxidizing system found in many tissues, helped greatly to advance knowledge concerning the mechanism of action of these substances. Extensive studies *in vivo* proved the value of BAL in reducing greatly the toxicity and in hastening the excretion not only of compounds of arsenic but also of mercury and certain other elements. A highly water-soluble dithiol of low toxicity, the O-glycoside of BAL, was tested by Danielli and colleagues (15), but technical difficulties of preparation in a form suitable for human therapy so far have prevented its general use.

The space devoted to this now historical development is regarded as entirely appropriate, since the general implications of these findings justified much optimism concerning the future of the metabolic approach to the development of chemotherapeutic agents. It was indicated that as sufficient knowledge is accumulated concerning essential metabolic pathways and intermediates, possibilities for logically influencing living processes may become evident. Also, new evidence was provided that even partial explanations of the mechanism of action of agents (e.g., arsenicals), whose biological activity had been disclosed empirically, could be of fundamental importance to chemotherapeutic advance.

III. THE ANTIMETABOLITE CONCEPT

The importance of a metabolic explanation of the mechanism of action of a drug saw its fullest application in the development of the theory of the mechanism of action of p-aminobenzene-sulfonamide (sulfanilamide) and its derivatives as competitive antagonists of the utilization by microorganisms of p-aminobenzoic acid (PABA). Although the functions of PABA in bacterial metabolism have been only partly clarified, enough became evident almost immediately following the work of Woods in 1940 (62), that Fildes in the same year was able to make his now famous prediction concerning the possibility of developing new chemotherapeutic agents by structural alteration of known metabolites (24). Observations of the antagonistic activity of certain analogues of naturally occurring substances had been made two years earlier by Dyer (16) and by Woolley and his associates (66), but it was the relationship between sulfonamides and PABA that focused attention on this new concept.

During subsequent years vigorous efforts have been made to find new chemotherapeutic agents through the deliberate chemical alteration of many compounds of importance to various forms of life. From these investigations, which have been reviewed many times during the last ten years (61, 56, 63, 64, 65), there has emerged a considerable body of information concerning the types of structural variation which are likely to be valuable in the design of antimetabolites. Also, many compounds of great biological activity have been obtained, and some of these have proved to be of considerable importance as tools for the study of metabolic processes. But, of valuable chemotherapeutic agents derived as a result of this concept, there has indeed been a paucity.

Until recently the compounds designed for use as antimetabolites have been, for the most part, analogues of cofactor-precursors essential to the life of mammals, and it is not surprising, therefore, that many of these are toxic to animals which are dependent upon the metabolites that the analogues resemble. A further complication that soon became apparent in the study of antimetabolites was the finding that analogues are most likely to be effective when the requirement of the organism for the corresponding metabolite must be satisfied exogenously.

A basis for this latter phenomenon perhaps is to be found in the use by different organisms of more than one mechanism (utilizing different intermediates) for the synthesis of each cofactor or other "multiple-component molecule." If a precursor must be supplied exogenously, or if an intermediate in one of these mechanisms of synthesis is closely similar in certain physicochemical properties to an analogue (which is able to reach the site of conversion of the intermediate), an opportunity is afforded for antagonistic activity to be exerted by the analogue. On the other hand, another organism may utilize a different pathway of biosynthesis of the same cofactor, with the involvement of intermediates that actually are quite different from the "analogue" in physicochemical properties, and for such organisms the "analogue" should have little or no inhibitory activity. Certainly, in cases where the pathway of biosynthesis of an important metabolite in an organism is unknown, it is not possible to design antimetabolic analogues with any degree of certainty.

It might be suggested that sulfonamides are effective inhibitors of many microorganisms that need no external supply of PABA because a compound identical with or very closely resembling PABA actually appears as an obligatory intermediate in the development of the cell. On the other hand, the fact that the sulfonic-acid analogue of pantothenic acid (pantoyltaurine) suppresses the growth of organisms which need an external supply of pantothenic acid, but is unable to block the growth of bacteria that have no such requirement, suggests that these latter organisms may synthesize coenzyme A (or a similar substance) from intermediates that do not include pantothenic acid, as such. However, a related analogue (e.g., phenylpantothenone), which inhibits not only organisms that must obtain the vitamin from their environment, but also others without such a requirement, may have the ability to block the utilization not only of pantothenic acid, but also of a related intermediate, which differs from pantothenic acid, but is used in the synthesis of a coenzyme A-like substance by certain organisms. These views, though speculative, may help to focus attention on one of the many problems encountered in the "antimetabolite approach" to the design of effective antagonists.

Because of the complications discussed, and others, and the failure until recently of the antimetabolite approach to chemotherapy to produce outstandingly effective new drugs, there has been a tendency on the part of some to disparage the antimetabolite concept. This seems rather shortsighted, when it is considered that the therapeutic success of the sulfonamide antagonists of PABA is dependent primarily on the fact that mammals have no apparent metabolic requirement for this important bacterial intermediary metabolite. Obviously we need to discover other compounds which, though essential to the metabolism of parasitic invaders, are of no importance to the host, or, at least, of much less importance to the host than to the parasite. Despite much investigation in fields likely to disclose such metabolic distinctions, the differences which have been turned up so far are, for the most part, quantitative rather than qualitative in nature. Accordingly, let us consider what can be done with only quantitative differences in requirement as a basis for scientific advance along the antimetabolite pathway.

IV. ANTAGONISTS OF THE "FOLIC-ACID SYSTEM"

1. The "4-Amino Analogues" of Folic Acid

Until recently the only outstanding examples of therapeutically useful antimetabolites, other than the sulfonamides, have been those compounds closely related to pteroylglutamic acid (folic acid) which contain an amino group in place of the hydroxyl group in position-4, in particular "Aminopterin" and "A-methopterin."

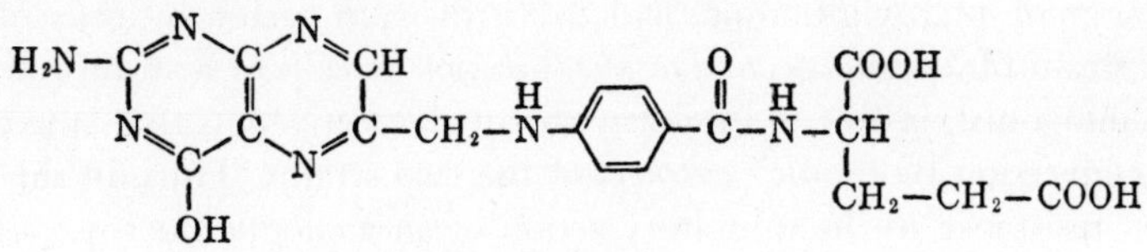

Pteroylglutamic acid

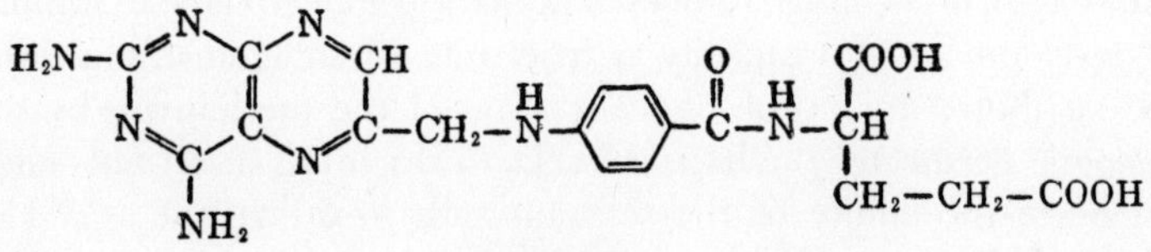

"Aminopterin"

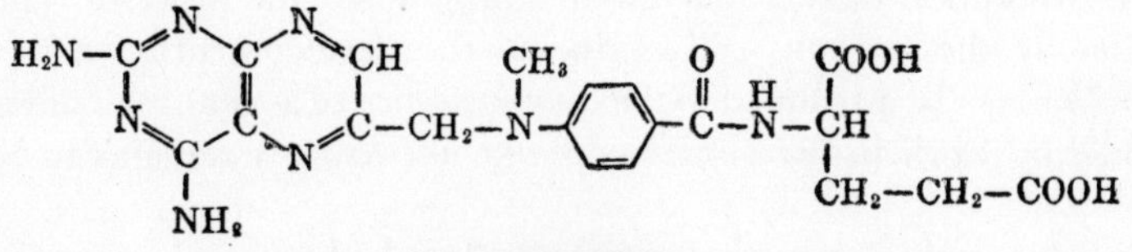

"A-methopterin"

FIG. 1.

Even before the significance of folic acid was established, with respect to the biosynthesis of derivatives of purine, thymine, serine, methionine, and other metabolites, it became evident that derivatives of folic acid are importantly involved in hematopoiesis. Accordingly, many analogues of folic acid were prepared and those mentioned above soon found an important place in the chemotherapy of leukemia, particularly in the temporary suppression of the acute leukemia of children (23). Although active also in suppressing certain other neoplastic processes, and widely employed today, many limitations on the use of these compounds have been encountered. One limitation is the rather delicate adjustment that must be maintained between maximal attainable inhibition of the formation of abnormal leucocytes and the appearance of highly undesirable effects attributable to the inhibition of normal cellular activities that also are dependent on a cofactor derived from folic acid.

Of even greater significance, however, is the fact that only about half of the cases treated with these antagonists respond, and in these originally susceptible individuals the remissions are not maintained. Both in bacteria (10) and in mouse leukemia there is now convincing evidence that loss of susceptibility to "A-methopterin" is attributable to the chemical selection of spontaneously occurring resistant mutant strains (9, 43).

More will be said subsequently concerning resistance to chemotherapeutic agents; however, it should be noted here that Nichol and associates demonstrated (49) that "A-methopterin," which inhibits the enzymatic conversion of pteroylglutamic acid to citrovorum factor by cells of the parent strain of *Streptococcus faecalis,* but not by cells of a strain resistant to the antagonist, is able to inhibit with equal effectiveness the same enzymatic conversion by "sonic" *extracts* of the two strains. Thus, in this case at least, resistance to the inhibitory action of an analogue does not appear to be attributable to the often-suggested circumvention of the need for an enzyme system, or a change in the susceptibility of an enzyme to inhibition, or the development of a capacity to inactivate an antagonist, but rather it may be attributed to a profound alteration of the mechanism by which the analogue permeates the bacterial cells to reach the susceptible enzyme system. Since the ability of the resistant cells to utilize the very closely related metabolite, pteroylglutamic acid, is not diminished, it would appear that the absorption of the analogue is a highly specific process. Whether exclusion by the resistant cell is due to the development of a type of "barrier" or is to be attributed to the disappearance of a "binding" substance (as stated by Ehrlich, *"corpora non agunt nisi fixata"*) remains to be explained.

In the similarly "A-methopterin"-resistant leukemia of mice it was found by Nichol that the concentration of the analogue required to inhibit the enzyme system (of the intact resistant cells) which forms citrovorum factor from folic acid is only about four times higher than that required for the parent strain (46, 48). Proof that this difference is sufficient to explain the escape of leukemic processes from inhibition *in vivo* is not yet available. However, it is not unlikely that such will prove to be the case, for a reduction of this magnitude in the transport of the antagonist to the sensitive enzyme system within the resistant leukemic cells should permit their reproductive processes to progress at a rate approaching that of un-treated leukemic tissue. It will be obvious that the susceptibility of normal tissues to inhibition prevents the concentration of the antagonists from being increased sufficiently to overcome even the moderate diminution in sensitivity which was observed.

Although it has not yet been established that the development of re-sistance to analogues of folic acid in originally susceptible human leukemias has a similar explanation, it would seem reasonable to anticipate that this is the case. It is conceivable that the "permeability" of leukemic cells of patients who are insusceptible *initially* to these analogues may closely resemble that of the chemically selected resistant mutants, with respect to behavior in the presence of the 4-amino analogues of folic acid. However, further work will be needed to determine whether or not this is true.

It is of considerable interest that from "A-methopterin"-sensitive forms of mouse leukemia, a strain has been evolved by Law (42) in which the analogue *hastens* the development of the abnormal cells, and on which citrovorum factor has a detectable inhibitory effect. Although a metabolic explanation of this remarkable development of partial dependence on "A-methopterin" has not been provided, it has been shown (48) that the dependent leukemia does not have the capacity to overproduce the citro-vorum factor, in a manner resembling the situation encountered in an "A-methopterin"-resistant strain of *S. faecalis* (3, 49) [or similar to that observed, with respect to PABA, in a sulfonamide-dependent strain of *Neurospora* (20, 68)]. Using streptomycin-dependent *E. coli,* Goldstein (28) recently has been able to demonstrate that, almost certainly, depend-ence, like resistance, results from a chance mutation and is not induced by the drug.

2. 2,4-Diaminopyrimidines as Antagonists of the "Folic-acid System"

It will be appropriate now to give attention to important chemothera-peutic advances which have resulted from extensive studies, by Hitchings and his collaborators, of the metabolic requirements of certain micro-organisms, particularly *Lactobacillus casei* and *Streptococcus faecalis.* These many investigations, which constitute a landmark in the metabolic approach to chemotherapy, offer a wealth of information concerning the structural requirements for interference with the purine, pyrimidine, and pteroylglutamic-acid metabolism of these organisms. Among other things it was shown, for example, that many derivatives of 2,4-diaminopyrimidine (including certain 2,4-diaminopteridines) are able profoundly to interfere with the function of folic acid or its metabolic derivatives.

While these investigations were in progress, extensive studies of a new antimalarial, chloroguanide ("Paludrine"), were in progress in various parts of the world. This compound, which had been developed by Curd, Davey, and Rose (14) in England in 1945, on the basis of empirical findings (and, as the authors have indicated, in spite of, rather than because of, theories concerning the relation of chemical structure to antimalarial activity) was a new departure from the important conventional derivatives of acridine or the aminoquinolines with antimalarial activity. After considerable study of chloroguanide two very interesting facts concerning it emerged: one, it is not active until it has been altered metabolically [Hawking and Perry (34)] (Fig. 2), and two, its biological activity is antagonized by folic acid (21). Although examination of its structure, as usually presented, suggests no obvious explanation for this unexpected result, Hitchings was able to deduce that the compound formed may be regarded as a triazine analogue of the 2,4-diaminopyrimidines (Fig. 2), many of which had been found capable of functioning as antagonists of the folic-acid system.

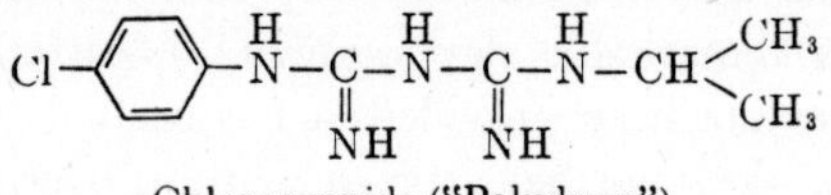

Chloroguanide ("Paludrine")

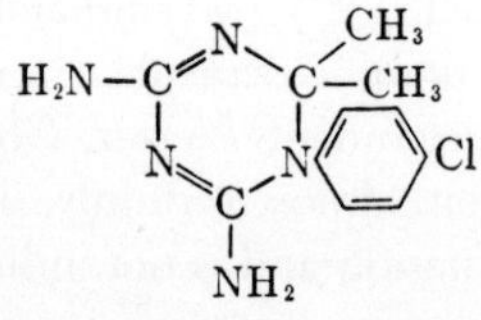

Chloroguanide metabolite 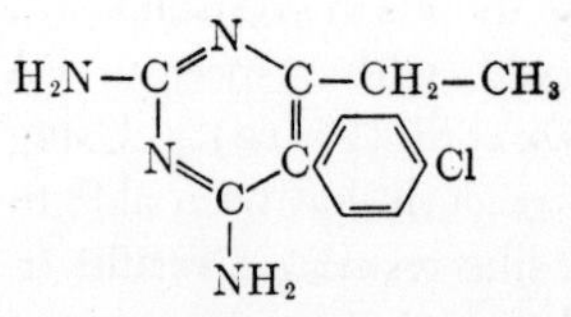   Pyrimethamine ("Daraprim")

FIG. 2.

Thus, it appears that the antimalarial activity of chloroguanide may be dependent on its serving as a precursor of an inhibitor of the utilization by plasmodia of compounds of the "folic-acid series." Additional evidence in favor of this possibility was afforded by the fact that certain malarial plasmodia are known to require p-aminobenzoic acid, in fact some species are quite susceptible to inhibition by various derivatives of sulfanilamide.

In the meantime, Hitchings and his colleagues, having surveyed their results with the various 2,4-diaminopyrimidine antagonists of the folic-acid system of bacteria, carried out an extensive synthetic program which was guided by what Hitchings has referred to appropriately as "enlightened empiricism." As a result, certain key compounds with very marked anti-metabolite activity for bacteria were chosen for testing against various experimental infections, among them malaria (38, 21a). In fact, it has been stated that the feeling of the investigators at this stage was, "We have a chemotherapeutic weapon; let us now see what infections we can cure with it."

The data relating chemical structure to biological activity that have been accumulated from these studies are impressive, and justify much more attention than can be devoted to them here. In essence, the highest potencies were found when 2,4-diaminopyrimidine was substituted in position-5 with a group such as phenyl and, with substitution of the benzene ring with a chlorine atom in the para-position (or, even better, with a second chlorine in the meta-position) the activity was increased further; also a small alkyl group was desirable in position-6. It must suffice to state here that, of the many compounds studied, the one with the greatest therapeutic advantage for use in the chemotherapy of malaria appeared to be pyrimethamine ("Daraprim") (Fig. 2). The similarity of the structure of this compound to that of the metabolite of chloroguanide is indeed most remarkable. This new chemotherapeutic agent has already been used widely and appears to have a promising future in the prophylaxis and treatment of various forms of malaria. Since, in the doses recommended for clinical use, e.g., 25 mg once per week, no signs of toxic effects of any kind have been reported, this new compound stands in sharp contrast to such antimalarials as quinacrine (atabrine) of World War II and its many successors. Probably pyrimethamine will be used principally as a suppressive in malaria, rather than for therapy of acute attacks, since its effects develop less rapidly than do those of chloroquine, a 4-amino-quinoline derivative which (in some cases together with the 8-amino-quinoline, primaquine) seems to offer the most favorable opportunity for a rapid cure following an acute attack of malaria. Pyrimethamine is active not only against the forms of the malaria parasite found in the blood, but also on the pre-erythrocytic forms of P. falciparum and, to a lesser extent, of P. vivax. Although gametocytes are not killed, it appears that they may be made unable to develop subsequently in mosquitoes (33).

The chief difficulty with pyrimethamine, as with chloroguanide, is the rapidity with which resistance can be developed by plasmodia. With chloroguanide the situation has now become serious, since the rather widespread use of this drug, in doses insufficient to cure, apparently has resulted in the development of highly resistant strains, particularly in certain parts of Africa. Although with pyrimethamine the problem of resistance is much less critical, because its activity is much higher than that of chloroguanide, a real difficulty is offered by the cross-resistance between the two agents. Thus, resistance to pyrimethamine may develop rapidly in strains of plasmodia which have been exposed to chloroguanide. It is worth noting that a significant degree of resistance is *not* observed with the important antimalarials derived from 4-amino-quinoline (e.g., chloroquine) and 8-amino-quinoline (e.g., primaquine).

The very marked tendency of mutant cells of various forms of life (e.g., bacteria, plasmodia, neoplastic leucocytes) to possess profound resistance to derivatives of 2,4-diaminopyrimidine (including "Aminopterin" and "A-methopterin") is in need of explanation. Because of the structural relationship and the similar mechanism of action of compounds of the pyrimethamine type and the 4-amino analogues of folic acid, it might be expected that a considerable degree of cross-resistance between the two series would be found. However, Hutchison and Burchenal, using a profoundly "A-methopterin"-resistant strain of *Leuconostoc citrovorum,* found that the sensitivity to the dichloro compound related to pyrimethamine [i.e., 2,4-diamino-5(3'4'-dichlorophenyl)-6-methylpyrimidine] was reduced concomitantly by only about 10-fold (39). With a strain of *S. faecalis* markedly resistant to "A-methopterin" (3,000,000-fold increase in resistance), the concomitant decrease in susceptibility to the dichloro compound was only about 250-fold (10). The reverse situation was somewhat more striking: the susceptibility to "A-methopterin" of a strain of *S. faecalis* very markedly resistant to the dichloro compound was decreased simultaneously by about 10,000-fold (11). Thus, it would appear that the development of a "barrier" to the utilization of one inhibitor has a variable influence on the susceptibility to the other, and certainly does not lead (in these species) to an equivalent loss in susceptibility to each type of inhibitor.

The similarity in the mechanisms of action of the two classes of compounds might suggest that those of the "A-methopterin" type also should have antimalarial activity. However, this application of these substances would appear to be precluded by their great affinity for various susceptible host cells, e.g., those of the hematopoietic and gastro-intestinal tissues. That such variations in chemical structure do permit a considerable degree of pharmacological specificity, so that "anti-folics" can be used in two quite different ways, justifies continued hope for further advances in specificity and clinical utility.

Although the 4-amino analogues of folic acid have much more affinity for certain tissues of animals than is the case with compounds of the pyrimethamine type, the latter are by no means lacking in this quality. Thus, pyrimethamine is able to produce severe and progressive intoxication when administered in relatively large amounts, and the related-dichloro compound is very much more active in this respect (57, 45). It has been shown in rats that this toxic effect, which appears to involve an inhibition of the utilization of derivatives of folic acid, cannot be as effectively reversed by the metabolically active derivative of folic acid, citrovorum factor (folinic acid), as by a substance in liver. On the other hand, the inhibitory activity for *S. faecalis* is readily reversed by citrovorum factor, but not by folic acid. It may be concluded that these compounds, as do the 4-amino derivatives of folic acid (47, 3a), interfere with the conversion of folic acid to citrovorum factor and, in animals, with the subsequent utilization of the latter (37).

The close similarity between the mechanisms of action of compounds of the pyrimethamine group and those of the chloroguanide class is indicated also by the finding that, as with the pyrimidine derivatives, the addition (in the meta-position) of a second chlorine atom to the phenyl ring of the metabolite of chloroguanide also produces a compound with much greater antimalarial (and toxic) activity (33). Work by Modest, Foley, Farber, and their associates (44, 22, 25, 26, 27) on a large group of 1,2-dihydro-*s*-triazines active as inhibitors of *S. faecalis* (and also, on a temporary basis, of certain forms of leukemia) led to an independent choice (25) of a dichloro compound identical with the above-mentioned derivative of chloroguanide.

In patients with acute leukemia, neither pyrimethamine nor the related dichloro-(pyrimidine)-derivative has proved to be as useful as the 4-amino analogues of folic acid (45). With the dichloro compound there was a higher incidence of undesirable side-effects (which closely resemble those produced by "A-methopterin") at dosage levels necessary for therapeutic results to be obtained. Also, the duration of these effects, following withdrawal of the drug, was more prolonged with the dichloro compound than with the pteridine derivative. It was demonstrated, in one patient, that the effects of the dichloro compound on the bone marrow could be prevented by the simultaneous administration of leucovorin (synthetic citrovorum factor) (45).

Another compound, which can be regarded as a derivative of 2,4-diaminopyrimidine and is of considerable biological interest, is 2,6-diaminopurine. This compound, which produced selective effects on neoplastic cells in tissue culture (2) and on certain experimental solid tumors, has not proved to be especially useful in man, although it has been shown by Burchenal and his associates to be active in prolonging the survival time of leukemic mice (6, 7). The status of this compound as a possible intermediate (or derivative of one) in the conversion of adenine to guanine remains to be clarified (1).

V. 6-MERCAPTOPURINE

A quite different type of compound, which may be regarded as another important product of the metabolic studies of Hitchings and his associates with microorganisms, is 6-mercaptopurine, the formula of which (together with that of adenine) is shown in Fig. 3.

$$
\begin{array}{cc}
\text{N}=\text{C}-\text{NH}_2 & \text{N}=\text{C}-\text{SH} \\
\text{HC}\quad\text{C}-\text{NH}{\scriptstyle\searrow}\text{CH} & \text{HC}\quad\text{C}-\text{NH}{\scriptstyle\searrow}\text{CH} \\
\text{N}-\text{C}-\text{N} & \text{N}-\text{C}-\text{N} \\
\text{Adenine} & \text{6-Mercaptopurine}
\end{array}
$$

Fig. 3.

This compound was shown to be a potent inhibitor of the growth of *L. casei* and to interfere with its metabolism of purines; although its activity for *L. casei* is prevented by adenine, guanine, hypoxanthine, or xanthine, none of these or other compounds, alone or in combination, is able to counteract the toxic effects of the analogue in animals (17, 18). With it, Clarke and his associates (12, 13) were able not only to inhibit the growth of sarcoma 180, but also to obtain *permanent* regression in a significant proportion of these tumors. In mice with transplanted leukemia, a prolongation of survival time has been obtained with strains either sensitive or resistant to "A-methopterin."

The use of this compound in the treatment of leukemia and allied diseases of man has been studied most extensively by Burchenal and his group and a report describing their results recently has become available (8). In general, the clinical and hematologic findings obtained were similar to those seen with the analogues of folic acid. About two-thirds (43) of a group of 68 children with acute leukemia responded initially to the purine analogue; in 29 of these the clinical and hematologic remissions were considered to be good. A much smaller proportion of remissions was obtained in a group of (50) adult individuals with acute leukemia, but here the frequency of induced remissions was appreciably higher than has been observed with the analogues of folic acid (8, 5). In chronic myelocytic leukemia remissions have been obtained in both early and late stages. In fact, of 10 cases of chronic myelocytic leukemia in early stages, all have responded to 6-mercaptopurine, a result apparently unparalleled in previous experiences with antimetabolites [Burchenal (5)].

Unfortunately, resistance to 6-mercaptopurine soon develops in acute leukemia, as is the case with the analogues of folic acid; in fact, the available evidence suggests that resistance to 6-mercaptopurine appears even more rapidly than with the folic-acid derivatives. However, the activity of the compound appears to bear no relation to the presence or absence of a state of resistance to "A-methopterin."

VI. THE POSSIBILITIES OF POTENTIATION AND THE AVOIDANCE OF RESISTANCE

The finding that there is no cross-resistance between 6-mercaptopurine and the 4-amino analogues of folic acid indicates not only that the use of the one substance following the other might permit a further brief prolongation of life in susceptible cases of acute leukemia, but, much more hopefully, that a means of circumventing resistance might be afforded through the simultaneous use of a combination of such agents. Through such an approach the development of a strain of drug-resistant mutants conceivably might be avoided: with the right combination of chemotherapeutic agents, where independent mechanisms of action are involved and cross-resistance is not found, the one drug might inhibit the resistant mutants left by the other.

Although Skipper and his associates (58) observed some potentiation of the activity of "A-methopterin" through the simultaneous administration of 6-mercaptopurine, in that there was an increase in the time of survival of mice with leukemia (L-1210) treated with the combination as compared with the effects obtained with either drug alone, the fatality of the disease was not altered. Unfortunately, the results so far obtained in acute leukemia treated with the same combination also have been disappointing.

The reason for this essential failure should be determined, since no real hope for successful chemotherapy of even this form of neoplasia can be hoped for, on the basis of present knowledge, until a means of preventing the survival of drug-resistant mutants can be found. However, it should be realized that the failure of this combination to cure leukemia, particularly in mice, probably is *not* to be attributed solely to the selection of resistant variants. It is a manifestation also of the incomplete inhibition of the proliferation of leukemia cells which is possible with these agents, because of the limitation on dosage imposed by the profound need of normal cells for the metabolites to which the analogues correspond. It is true, of course, that selection of resistant mutants is made possible by the fact that the drugs now available are not sufficiently potent to permit, under the conditions of their usage, adequate suppression of proliferative mechanisms within all neoplastic cells of a given population.

Let us examine a few other interesting examples of potentiation through the use of combination therapy. Although, as might be expected, pyrimethamine and the related dichloro compound show only additive effects as inhibitors of *L. casei*, the activity of pyrimethamine is markedly potentiated by the purine analogue, 6-mercaptopurine; similarly, the activity of pyrimethamine as an inhibitor of *S. faecalis* is markedly potentiated by 6-azathymine (19). This analogue of thymine, which also has been studied extensively in our laboratories (52, 53, 54), is of considerable interest and will be treated later.

Thymine   6-Azathymine

FIG. 4.

Another interesting example of potentiation is to be found in the inhibitory actions of 6-azathymine and 8-azaguanine on *S. faecalis* (19).

Metabolic studies such as these, although making use of bacterial "models," can be regarded as offering renewed hope that continued investigation may lead to greater chemotherapeutic success. Even though 8-azaguanine has not lived up to the flurry that accompanied the announcement of its chemotherapeutic activity against certain cancers in mice (41), its study contributed very significantly to the realization of the important fact that selective inhibition of the growth of cancer tissue is possible. Furthermore, a sound metabolic explanation for the inactivity of azaguanine against many tumors in mice, and in man, has been afforded by the demonstration of the rapid enzymatic conversion of azaguanine to an inactive derivative by most neoplastic and many normal human tissues (35).

6-Azathymine, as such, presumably will not be able to interfere with mammalian metabolic reactions, since thymine, the naturally occurring base which it resembles, is utilized anabolically by normal tissues to only a very slight degree (51, 4, 38); however, the type of activity exerted on certain microorganisms encourages the study of its desoxyriboside in mammalian tissues. Although it is a competitive antagonist of the utilization of both thymine and its desoxyriboside (thymidine) by *S. faecalis* under ordinary conditions, a most interesting situation is encountered when a resistant mutant of this organism develops in the presence of "Aminopterin." Under these conditions, 6-azathymine profoundly inhibits the growth of the mutant cells; in fact, the inhibition appears not to be reversed by thymidine after a brief exposure to the analogue (Hakala *et al.*, 32). That the irreversible inhibition of growth results from an incorporation of the analogue into desoxyribonucleic acid is as yet only an hypothesis, albeit an attractive one. The possibility of obtaining a similar effect on mammalian cells undergoing reproduction, under those conditions of minimal synthesis of functional derivatives of thymine which should be obtainable by the simultaneous administration of "Aminopterin," has been considered to be sufficiently attractive to justify the preparation of the desoxyriboside of 6-azathymine. Although chemical synthesis cannot be accomplished at the present time, the compound has now been prepared biologically (Prusoff, 53), by a transdesoxyribosidation reaction. It will be appreciated, of course, that the pathways of anabolic utilization of thymidine by mammalian cells may not sufficiently resemble those of such organisms as *S. faecalis* as to permit "azathymidine" to function in the way so hopefully indicated by bacterial studies; however, data on this point should be available soon.

Another development of theoretical interest, which may be mentioned briefly, is the preparation of an antagonist of orotic acid (29, 30, 31) (Fig. 5).

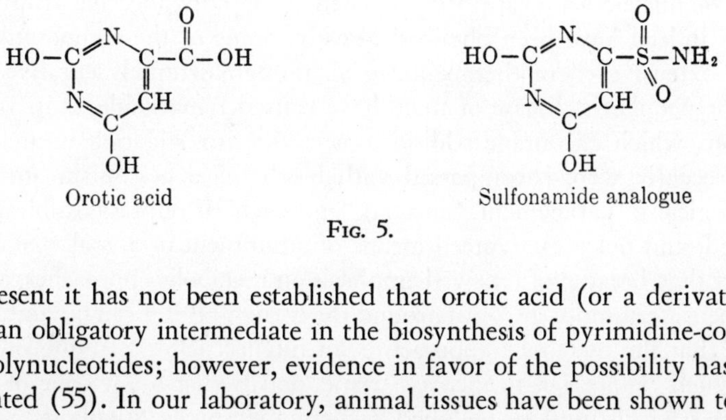

Orotic acid   Sulfonamide analogue

Fig. 5.

At present it has not been established that orotic acid (or a derivative of it) is an obligatory intermediate in the biosynthesis of pyrimidine-containing polynucleotides; however, evidence in favor of the possibility has been presented (55). In our laboratory, animal tissues have been shown to contain an enzyme system which utilizes orotic acid and forms uridine-5-phosphate without the intermediate formation of uracil. This has been established by the use of orotic acid labeled with C^{14} either in position-2 or in the carboxyl group (Karger and Carter, 40). Although only preliminary tests of the orotic-acid analogue, 2,4-dihydroxy-6-sulfonamide-pyrimidine, have so far been possible in this system, the new antagonist has proved to be an effective inhibitor of the utilization of orotic acid by it, as well as by a strain of *Lactobacillus bulgaricus* 09 which requires an exogenous supply of orotic acid. Since the corresponding sulfonic acid analogue is quite inactive, it is conceivable that analogues of even higher activity can be obtained by appropriate substitutions of the amide-nitrogen and the preparation of such derivatives is now in progress.

VII. FINAL CONSIDERATIONS

In spite of encouraging results with inhibitors of the synthesis of compounds required, so far as is known, by all cells, it must be emphasized that greater hope must be held for chemotherapeutic agents that block the utilization of compounds of specific importance to parasitic invaders whether these be bacterial, protozoal, viral, or neoplastic. In order to attain this goal metabolic investigation of all varieties of disease-producing entities must be prosecuted vigorously. It is encouraging, for example, to learn from the investigations of Wyatt and Cohen (67) that the desoxyribonucleic acid of certain bacteriophages contains hydroxymethylcytosine in place of all cytosine. Surely this fundamental difference is the type of "lead" that is needed if chemotherapy is to be put on an increasingly rational basis and an opportunity for really profound effects on invading cells or organisms is to be found.

In conclusion, then, it is evident that metabolic approaches to chemotherapy, especially in areas which may yield specific inhibitors of the synthesis of nucleic acids, are being opened up rapidly and that stimulating results indeed have been obtained already. Some of the compounds now under extensive chemotherapeutic trial, though definitely curative of no viral or neoplastic disease of man, have caused remarkable temporary remissions which encourage additional scientific investigation in areas that until recently were encompassed with biochemical pessimism and pharmacological disparagement. Since an "approach" is only a possible way to proceed, and not a guaranteed means of attainment of a goal, one cannot predict that, because of renewed emphasis on metabolic approaches, chemotherapeutic triumphs are "just around the corner." But it can be confidently stated that the metabolic approach is an intellectually satisfying one, and one which cannot fail to increase tremendously that knowledge of living processes which must be obtained if chemotherapy eventually is to escape from the state of contented empiricism in which, until recently, it has been submerged.

REFERENCES

1. Bendich, A., Furst, S. S., and Brown, G. B. (1950). *J. Biol. Chem.* 185, 423.
2. Biesele, J. J., Berger, R. E., Wilson, A. Y., Hitchings, G. H., and Elion, G. B. (1951). *Cancer* 4, 186.
3. Broquist, H. P., Kohler, A. R., Hutchison, D. J., and Burchenal, J. H. (1953). *J. Biol. Chem.* 202, 59.

3a. Broquist, H. P., Stokstad, E. L. R., and Jukes, T. H. (1950). *J. Biol. Chem.* 185, 399.

4. Brown, G. B., Roll, P. M., and Weinfeld, H. (1952). *in* Phosphorus Metabolism ed. by W. D. McElroy and B. Glass, Vol. 2, p. 388. The Johns Hopkins Press, Baltimore.

5. Burchenal, J. H. (1954). Personal communication.

6. Burchenal, J. H., Bendich, A., Brown, G. B., Elion, G. B., Hitchings, G. H., Rhoads, C. P., and Stock, C. C. (1949). *Cancer* 2, 119.

7. Burchenal, J. H., Karnofsky, D. A., Kingsley-Pillers, E. M., Southam, C. M., Myers, W. P. L., Escher, G. C., Craver, L. F., Dargeon, H. W., and Rhoads, C. P. (1951). *Cancer* 4, 549.

8. Burchenal, J. H., Murphy, M. L., Ellison, R. R., Sykes, M. P., Tan, T. C., Leone, L. A., Karnofsky, D. A., Craver, L. F., Dargeon, H. W., and Rhoads, C. P. (1953). *Blood* 8, 965.

9. Burchenal, J. H., Robinson, E., Johnston, S. F., and Kushida, M. N. (1950). *Science* 111, 116.

10. Burchenal, J. H., Waring, G. B., and Hutchison, D. J. (1951). *Proc. Soc. Exptl. Biol. Med.* 78, 311.

11. Burchenal, J. H., Waring, G. B., and Hutchison, D. J. (1953). *Proc. Soc. Exptl. Biol. Med.* 82, 536.

12. Clarke, D. A., Philips, F. S., Sternberg, S. S., Stock, C. C., and Elion, G. B. (1953). *Proc. Am. Assoc. Can. Research* 1, 9.

13. Clarke, D. A., Philips, F. S., Sternberg, S. S., Stock, C. C., Elion, G. B., and Hitchings, G. H. (1953). 13, 593.

14. Curd, F. H. S., Davey, D. G., and Rose, F. L. (1945). *Ann. Trop. Med. Parisitol.* 39, 157.

15. Danielli, J. F., Danielli, M., Fraser, J. B., Mitchell, P. D., Owen, L. N., and Shaw, G. (1947). *Biochem. J.* 41, 325.

16. Dyer, H. M. (1938). *J. Biol. Chem.* 124, 519.

17. Elion, G. B., Burgi, E., and Hitchings, G. H. (1952). *J. Am. Chem. Soc.* 74, 411.

18. Elion, G. B., Hitchings, G. H., and VanderWerff, A. (1951). *J. Biol. Chem.* 192, 505.

19. Elion, G. B., Singer, S., and Hitchings, G. H. (1954). *J. Biol. Chem.* 208, 477.

20. Emerson, S. (1950). *Cold Spring Harbor Symposia Quant. Biol.* 14, 40.

21. Falco, E. A., Hitchings, G. H., Russell, P. B., and VanderWerff, H. (1949). *Nature* 164, 107.

21a. Falco, E. A., Goodwin, L. G., Hitchings, G. H., Rollo, I. M., and Russell, P. B. (1951). *Brit. J. Pharmacol.* 6, 185.

22. Farber, S., Diamond, I., Foley, G. E., and Modest, E. J. (1952). *Am. J. Path.* 28, 559.

23. Farber, S., Diamond, L. K., Mercer, R. D., Sylvester, R. F., Jr., and Wolff, J. A. (1948). *New Engl. J. Med.* 238, 787.

24. Fildes, P. (1940). *Lancet* i, 955.

25. Foley, G. E. (1953). *Proc. Soc. Exptl. Biol. Med.* 83, 733.

26. Foley, G. E. (1953). *Proc. Soc. Exptl. Biol. Med.* 83, 740.

27. Foley, G. E., and Watson, P. L. (1953). *Proc. Soc. Exptl. Biol. Med.* 83, 742.

28. Goldstein, A. (1954). Personal communication.

29. Greenbaum, S. B. (1954). To be published.

30. Greenbaum, S. B. and Holmes, W. L. (1954). *Abstr. 125th Meetings, Am. Chem. Soc.* (Kansas City, March 26), p. 31 N.

31. Greenbaum, S. B. and Holmes, W. L. (1954). *J. Am. Chem. Soc.* 76, 2899.
32. Hakala, M., Prusoff, W. H., and Welch, A. D. (1954). *Federation Proc.* 13, 223.
33. Hawking, F. (1953). Symposium on Growth Inhibition and Chemotherapy, VI Internat. Cong. of Microbiol., p. 88.
34. Hawking, F. and Perry, W. L. M. (1948). *Brit. J. Pharmacol.* 3, 320.
35. Hirshberg, E., Kream, J., and Gellhorn, A. (1952). *Cancer Research* 12, 524.
36. Hitchings, G. H., Elion, G. B., Falco, E. A., Russell, P. B., Sherwood, M. B., and VanderWerff, H. (1950). *J. Biol. Chem.* 183, 1.
37. Hitchings, G. H., Falco, E. A., Elion, G. B., Singer, S., Waring, G. B., Hutchison, D. J., and Burchenal, J. H. (1952). *Arch. Biochem. and Biophys.* 40, 479.
38. Holmes, W. L., Prusoff, W. H., and Welch, A. D. (1954). *J. Biol. Chem.* In press.
39. Hutchison, D. J. and Burchenal, J. H. (1952). *Proc. Soc. Exptl. Biol. Med.* 80, 516.
40. Karger, B. and Carter, C. E. (1954). To be published.
41. Kidder, G. W., Dewey, V. C., and Parks, R. E., Jr. (1949). *Science* 109, 511.
42. Law, L. W. (1951). *Proc. Soc. Exptl. Biol. Med.* 77, 340.
43. Law, L. W. and Boyle, P. J. (1950). *Proc. Soc. Exptl. Biol. Med.* 74, 599.
44. Modest, E. J., Foley, G. E., Pechet, M. M., and Farber, S. (1952). *J. Am. Chem. Soc.* 74, 855.
45. Murphy, M. L., Ellison, R. R., Karnofsky, D. A., and Burchenal, J. H. (1954). *J. Clin. Invest.* In press.
46. Nichol, C. A. (1954). *J. Pharmacol.* 110, 40.
47. Nichol, C. A. and Welch, A. D. (1950). *Proc. Soc. Exptl. Biol. Med.* 74, 403.
48. Nichol, C. A. and Welch, A. D. (1953). A.A.A.S. Symposium on Antimetabolites and Cancer (Boston, Dec. 28). In press.
49. Nichol, C. A., Zakrzewski, S., and Welch, A. D. (1953). *Proc. Soc. Exptl. Biol. Med.* 83, 272.
50. Peters, R. A., Stocken, L. A., and Thompson, R. H. S. (1945). *Nature* 156, 616.
51. Plentl, A. A. and Schoenheimer, R. (1944). *J. Biol. Chem.* 153, 203.
52. Prusoff, W. H. (1952). *Federation Proc.* 11, 271.
53. Prusoff, W. H. (1953). *Federation Proc.* 12, 358.
54. Prusoff, W. H., Holmes, W. L., and Welch, A. D. *Cancer Research.* In press.
55. Reichard, P. (1952). *J. Biol. Chem.* 197, 391.
56. Roblin, R. O., Jr. (1946). *Chem. Revs.* 38, 255.
57. Schmidt, L. H., Hughes, H. B., and Schmidt, I. G. (1953). *J. Pharmacol.* 107, 92.
58. Skipper, H., Thomson, J. R., Elion, G. B., and Hitchings, G. H. (1954). *Cancer Research.* 14, 294.
59. Stocken, L. A. and Thompson, R. H. S. (1945). *Biochem. J.* 40, 535.
60. Voegtlin, C., Dyer, H. A., and Leonard, C. S. (1923). *Public Health Repts. U.S.* 38, 1882.
61. Welch, A. D. (1945). *Physiol. Revs.* 25, 687.
62. Woods, D. D. (1940). *Brit. J. Exptl. Pathol.* 21, 74.
63. Woolley, D. W. (1947). *Physiol. Revs.* 27, 308.
64. Woolley, D. W. (1947). *Ann. Rev. Biochem.* 16, 359.
65. Woolley, D. W. (1952). A Study of Antimetabolites. John Wiley & Sons, New York.
66. Woolley, D. W., Strong, F. M., Madden, R. J., and Elvehjem, C. A. (1938). *J. Biol. Chem.* 124, 715.
67. Wyatt, G. R. and Cohen, S. S. (1952). *Nature* 170, 1072.
68. Zalokar, M. (1950). *J. Bacteriol.* 60, 191.

METABOLIC FACTORS AFFECTING CHEMOTHERAPEUTIC RESPONSE

By BERNARD D. DAVIS,* U. S. Public Health Service, Tuberculosis Research Laboratory, Cornell University Medical College, New York, N. Y.

BEFORE DISCUSSING the topic presented in the title, I should like to say a few words about the usage of the term "chemotherapeutic." This term was introduced by Ehrlich to refer to agents that are directly and selectively toxic to parasitic cells, in contrast to pharmacological agents which act on host cells. We are tending increasingly to blur this useful distinction. The extension of the term "chemotherapy" to include drugs that act selectively on abnormal host cells (e.g., anticancer or antithyroid chemotherapy) may have sufficient justification. But if we apply the same term to all new drugs whose action is dramatic, or involves a known chemical mechanism, we shall be condemning the term "pharmacology" to gradual extinction. It would, of course, be in good company, resting in the Elysian fields of science along with such honored veterans as "demography" and "natural philosophy." But those who would advocate this change should first make sure that it offers real advantages—and I doubt that it does.

And now I should like to discuss briefly some metabolic factors that affect the response of a parasite to chemotherapy. Let us first consider factors that depend on the genetics of the parasite, and later pass on to others that depend on the environment provided by the host.

The fact that chemotherapy depends for its existence on disunities in biochemistry—on differences between host and parasite—has been emphasized. And it is well known that many antimetabolites that effectively inhibit microorganisms *in vitro* have been disappointing when tested *in vivo*, presumably because they interfere with reactions that are as essential for the host as they are for the parasite. This development led to a good deal of discouragement about the rational approach to chemotherapy offered by antimetabolites. Indeed, at one time I felt that only metabolites peculiar to microorganisms were likely to be useful models for synthesizing antimetabolites; and it was partly on the basis of this view that we undertook an extensive search, through the use of mutants, for unknown microbial

* Present address: Department of Pharmacology, New York University College of Medicine, New York 16, N. Y.

metabolites (1, 2). Several of these have, indeed, turned out to be peculiar to microorganisms [p-hydroxybenzoic acid, (2, 3, 4); shikimic acid and related intermediates of aromatic biosynthesis (5, 6)]; but their discovery has not led to chemotherapeutically valuable new antimetabolites.

I should now like to re-examine this question on the basis of the assumption that marked differences in susceptibility to a drug, which can be observed even between closely related microbial strains, would be expected to exist *a fortiori* between microbial and animal cells. And such differences in drug resistance would presumably be based on the same biochemical mechanisms in both classes of cells. It is therefore pertinent to consider whether mutations that lead to increased drug resistance in microorganisms involve a qualitative shift in the nature of a metabolic path. To be sure, when the problem of drug resistance first became prominent some years ago it was customary to ascribe this resistance to such a mechanism— i.e., to the development of an alternative metabolic path, by-passing the metabolite with which the drug competes but leading ultimately to an identical later product. However, it seems extremely unlikely, from what we now know about relations between genes and enzymes, that a single mutation could give rise to the several new enzymes that one would expect would be needed for such a development. I would therefore reserve judgment on the existence of such a mechanism.

In any case, even if such a by-passing of a previously essential metabolite can be produced by a mutation, this mechanism could hardly be the universal basis for the development of drug resistance. For most strains become highly resistant to most drugs only through a series of steps, each making a quantitatively small contribution to the resistance. Such a process seems incompatible with the development of an alternative path, involving a new substrate. It is compatible, however, with a number of other, less gross, changes in the physiology of the cell (7).

Dr. Welch has presented evidence in this Symposium for one such mechanism, namely, decreased accessibility of drug to enzyme. We have obtained evidence for another mechanism: production of an altered enzyme that still carries out the same reaction but is less susceptible to inhibition by the drug (7). We have been particularly sympathetic to the latter possibility because of the demonstration by Maas (8) and by Horowitz (9) that a mutation can give rise to another kind of qualitative alteration in an enzyme (an increase in its temperature sensitivity) without changing the nature of the reaction that it catalyzes. Incidentally, we might note that we have sought for more direct evidence for such changes in affinity of an enzyme for an inhibitor, but this search has been hampered by the fact that the hundreds of available antimetabolities are, with few exceptions, analogues of metabolites (e.g., amino acids, purines, vitamins) that are not substrates of known enzymatic reactions.

To get back to the problem of designing chemotherapeutics: the point I should like to emphasize is that if two strains of bacteria can differ markedly in susceptibility to a given drug, even though both possess the reaction with which that drug interferes, then similar differences might be expected to occur between host and parasite cells. It would therefore seem premature to give up the hope of finding chemotherapeutically effective antimetabolites by modelling them on metabolites that are essential for both host and parasite. Indeed, the selective toxicity recently achieved with analogues of purines, pyrimidines, and folic acids offers concrete support for this view.

And now let us consider the effect that the environment provided by the host exerts on the response of the parasite to chemotherapeutic agents. For this purpose it is advisable to distinguish between bacteriostatic and bactericidal agents.

With bacteriostatic agents chemotherapeutic action requires that metabolic antagonists of the drug should not be present, at least in effective concentrations, at the sites of infection. Here the case of the sulfonamides is particularly instructive, since their inhibitory action has been shown to be reversible at three different metabolic levels. In the first place, competitive antagonism by *p*-aminobenzoic acid could reverse their action, but fortunately this compound is not per se a metabolite in mammals and apparently is not present in their body fluids under ordinary circumstances. Secondly, since *p*-aminobenzoic acid functions by virtue of its incorporation into members of the folic-acid group, these compounds are theoretically capable of noncompetitively antagonizing the sulfonamides, and, in fact, do so with certain enterococci which are thereby rendered insusceptible to sulfonamide chemotherapy. However, the folic-acid compounds that are found in the mammal fortunately are inert for most bacteria, and hence do not interfere with sulfonamide chemotherapy. This inertness presumably depends either on inability of the compounds to penetrate the bacteria, or on some difference between the mammalian and the bacterial "brands" of folic acid. This problem has not been resolved.

Finally, it has long been known that sulfonamide inhibition could also be reversed noncompetitively by a group of products of folic-acid metabolism, including certain amino acids, a purine, and the pyrimidine thymine. Since the normal body fluids are known to contain a variety of amino acids, the explanation for the effectiveness of sulfonamides in these fluids might be that nucleic-acid components are not present in them. I know of no direct evidence on this point, but considerable light is shed on it by the interesting observations of Bacon and Burrows (10). These investigators studied the effect of a variety of auxotrophic mutations on the pathogenicity of a virulent strain of Salmonella for mice. Mutants requiring various amino acids were found to have retained full pathogenicity, while a mutant requiring a purine had lost all pathogenicity. With this strain, however, pathogenicity could be restored by injecting into the host the compound required by the mutant parasite. (Similar behavior was exhibited by a p-aminobenzoic acid auxotroph.) This result strongly suggests that purines (and probably pyrimidines) are not present in significant amounts in mammalian body fluids. This conclusion can be extended to include the purine ribosides and ribotides, since in our experience these compounds have been at least as active as free purines for all purine auxotrophs.

As a corollary of these observations, the release of nucleic-acid components would seem likely to be the major factor responsible for the well-known ineffectiveness of sulfonamides in areas of extensive tissue destruction, including purulent infections, burns, and large wounds.

And now let us consider the bactericidal drugs. Much less is known about their mode of action, and no specific metabolic antagonists have generously stepped forward to point out the site of primary attack. However, one can say a little about the influence of the metabolic state of the bacteria on the rate at which they are sterilized by these drugs. And a consideration of this problem is obviously of practical importance, since optimal chemotherapy with these drugs depends on not only suppression but also rapid eradication of the infecting parasites by the drug.

Penicillin, as is well known, sterilizes bacteria only under conditions that allow them to grow (11). Streptomycin has a less stringent requirement, but we have observed (12), as has Bryson (13), that this drug does require metabolic activity for optimal action. Thus streptomycin sterilizes E. coli cells very slowly in distilled water, buffer, or glucose solution, but many times as rapidly in a medium containing both phosphate and glucose. (The low rate in the incomplete medium presumably depends on endogenous metabolism.)

One can therefore conclude that a bacterial cell would not be sterilized by a drug either if it were sequestered in a location that prevented access of the drug, or if it were in a location that could not support the metabolic activity required for sterilization by the drug. The latter mechanism probably underlies the observation of Jawetz (14) that certain mixtures of bacteriostatic and bactericidal agents are chemotherapeutically less effective than the bactericidal agent alone.

One other metabolic factor suggests itself for consideration, which is not clearly either genetic or environmental in origin. I am referring to the phenomenon of "persisters" described by Bigger (15). When a population of bacteria is exposed to penicillin in the relatively homogeneous environment of a test tube, sterilization will proceed rapidly if the medium is adequate, but after some hours a small fraction of a percent of viable cells will be found to have survived, and these will persist for many hours more. Yet these cells are not drug-resistant in the ordinary sense, since on transfer to fresh medium without drug they give rise to clones of cells that are no more resistant to the drug than the original population. One is tempted to suggest that these "persisters" are in a metabolically dormant state, at least with respect to the metabolic reactions required for chemotherapy. And perhaps it is only a formal restatement of the problem to point out that these cells appear to be genotypically drug-sensitive but phenotypically drug-resistant. This is a difficult problem to investigate, since one cannot study such cells in large masses. However, it is clearly a problem of practical importance that deserves more investigation than it has received. And the investigation of such a discrepancy between genotype and phenotype might have important consequences for bacterial genetics and physiology. In this connection it might be noted that a well-defined discrepancy between genotype and phenotype has been observed among the products of a mixed infection with bacteriophage (16).

REFERENCES

1. Davis, B. D. (1950). *Experientia* 6, 41.
2. Davis, B. D. (1951). *J. Exptl. Med.* 94, 243.
3. Davis, B. D. (1950). *Nature* 166, 1120.
4. Snyder, J. C. and Davis, B. D. (1951). *Federation Proc.* 10, 419.
5. Davis, B. D. (1951). *J. Biol. Chem.* 191, 315.
6. Davis, B. D. (1952). *J. Bacteriol.* 64, 729.
7. Davis, B. D. and Maas, W. K. (1952). *Proc. Natl. Acad. Sci.* 38, 775.
8. Maas, W. K. and Davis, B. D. (1952). *Proc. Natl. Acad. Sci. U.S.* 38, 785.
9. Horowitz, N. H. and Fling, M. (1953). *Genetics* 38, 360.
10. Bacon, G. A., Burrows, T. W. and Yates, M. (1950). *Brit. J. Exptl. Pathol.* 31, 714.
11. Hobby, G. L., Meyer, K. and Chaffee, E. (1942). *Proc. Soc. Exptl. Biol. Med.* 50, 281.
12. Davis, B. D. (1948). *in* Bacterial and Mycotic Infections of Man, ed. by R. J. Dubos, p. 656. J. B. Lippincott, Philadelphia.
13. Bryson, V. Personal communication.
14. Jawetz, E., Gunnison, J. B., and Speck, R. S. (1951). *Am. J. Med. Sci.* 222, 404.
15. Bigger, J. W. (1944). *Lancet* ii, 497.
16. Novick, A. and Szilard, L. (1951). *Science* 113, 34.

COMPARATIVE BIOCHEMISTRY AND CHEMOTHERAPY

By Seymour S. Cohen, *The Children's Hospital of Philadelphia (Department of Pediatrics) and the Department of Physiological Chemistry, University of Pennsylvania Medical School*

This paper contains a discussion of comparative biochemistry as it affects the problem of developing a rational chemotherapy of infection.

At the present time "comparative biochemistry" is a poorly defined term that had at least two different interpretations in the last 20 years. We are all familiar with the excellent monograph of Baldwin which undertook, although concentrating on higher animals, to examine the biochemical processes associated with life in its most general sense. By examining many organisms and analyzing their similarities and differences, it was hoped that one might obtain clues concerning their evolution. As one notable success resulting from such an approach may be mentioned the studies of Meyerhof, Baldwin, etc. on the distribution of phosphagen in animal muscle, which have supported the theory of the evolution of the Chordata from the Echinodermata.

A number of other areas of exploration in this spirit have included research on blood-transport pigments, carotenoids and the A vitamins, bioluminescent substances, etc. The relations of nitrogenous excretion products and the organism's requirements in terms of salt and water balance have been studied in great detail. This subject has of necessity been concerned largely with the division of labor of many organs in the intact animal.

That there are metabolic differences, even among the Metazoa, is highlighted by this type of data, and it is not surprising, therefore, that biochemical differences have been employed in classification. For example, we may note that this approach to taxonomy has been of major importance in differentiating lichens. The tendency has been to regard chemically distinct individuals in this group as distant species, whether morphological differences are apparent or not. Indeed, the classification has reached a stage wherein the use of this approach for the analysis of fungus-algal consortia is stated by Lamb to be confusing the taxonomist, since biochemical variability has been found to exceed morphological and other types of more readily ascertainable variability.

Despite the evident importance of this type of comparative biochemistry to research in evolution, it is nonetheless true that this kind of investigation is not growing rapidly, for reasons which we need not explore at this time. Concurrent with the stasis or even decline of this school of comparative biochemistry has been the growth of an entirely independent school, formally begun by Kluyver and widely popularized by Van Niel and his students. From its inception, this group of microbiologists believed in the existence of common metabolic patterns and employed the phrase "the unity of biochemistry," a phrase which has been widely accepted in biochemical circles.[1] There is no question but that this working hypothesis has had major successes, as in the correlation of various growth factors and essential metabolites of microorganisms with coenzymatic function in higher organisms. However, it must be noted that, in the past, the orientation of this group has caused it to gloss over and to minimize some of the metabolic differences in various organisms. At the present time, however, the major proponents for the hypothesis of unity in biochemistry and, incidentally, for the corollary of a monophyletic development of organisms, are beginning to worry about the validity of their hypothesis. Van Niel has carefully remarked: "In the long run it may well be possible to get to the point where we say, 'Oh well, comparative biochemistry, there it is; it is much the same way in all organisms.' But we are not there yet."

On the other hand, proponents of a rational chemotherapy find it difficult to accept the rigorous formulation of the concept of "unity of biochemistry." Thus, it is held that chemotherapy exists only because the differential susceptibilities of host and parasite to a given inhibitor reflect important biochemical and metabolic differences between host and parasite. Furthermore, as Dr. Bueding has elegantly shown in his studies on the parasitic helminths, specific chemotherapy must take into account biochemical differences among parasites. This discussion will undertake to support and develop this orientation in comparative biochemistry, as important not only in understanding higher organisms but also in the analysis of metabolism at the single-cell level. A correct choice of outlook in comparative biochemistry is a matter of practical import, since our approach to this subject may help us in controlling infection.

It may be argued that the thesis of "the unity of biochemistry" holds in the main and that chemotherapy takes advantage of relatively minor variants in the large stream of metabolism. A quotation from Winston

[1] Probably the clearest definition of what is meant by the "unity of biochemistry" has been given by Wilson in discussing the data on nitrogen fixation:

"Although nature may make minor alterations to suit the convenience of a particular agent, the basic pattern of biological nitrogen fixation is essentially constant."

Churchill (taken out of context) will introduce some data against this argument: "In the problems which the Almighty sets His humble servants, things hardly ever happen the same way twice over, or if they seem to do so, there is some variant which stultifies undue generalization."

Let us indicate some of the kinds of biochemical variability which are already known. Organisms may display variability in their content of major components. Thus the tubercle bacillus, in contrast to the mammal, appears to contain:

a. Large amounts of D-arabinose, in the lipopolysaccharide in its cell wall.

b. α, ε-diaminopimelic acid, as a constituent of certain peptides.

c. Fatty acids containing cyclopropane rings.

d. Mycolic acids.

e. Phosphatides with amino acids other than serine.

It is conceivable that the biosynthesis of any one of these substances may provide a point of differential susceptibility to an inhibitor of appropriate configuration. We may mention further that tubercle bacillus does not appear to contain sterols, in contrast to the mammal.

In the same vein, it may be recalled that in the virus studies of Wyatt and the author, large amounts of a new pyrimidine, 5-hydroxymethyl cytosine, were discovered in a very limited group of bacterial viruses. This base has not been detected in *E. coli,* the host for these viruses, nor indeed in any other organisms as yet examined; virus, bacterium, plant, or animal.

The pyrimidine, 5-methylcytosine, found in plants and animals, has not yet been found in any virus or bacterium. If a bacterium wished to cure itself of a mammalian infection, it might well be advised to investigate the synthesis of this substance.

Organisms may vary in basic pathways for the synthesis of essential components. According to Davis, *E. coli* makes lysine via the decarboxylation of α, ε-diaminopimelic acid, whereas Neurospora and yeast are reported to convert α-aminoadipic acid to lysine. It is thought that lysine is essential for the mammal because the biosynthetic pathway for lysine was lost. But which biosynthetic pathway was lost? Or were both? This raises problems associated with the existence of multiple alternative pathways, which are becoming increasingly familiar to the biochemist.

Let us look at tryptophan degradation as an example. According to Stanier, there are at least three types of Pseudomonas strains which differ in the manner in which they degrade tryptophan. One group metabolizes the amino acid through the aromatic pathway via catechol, cis-cis muconic acid, etc., another through the quinoline pathway to kynurenic acid and perhaps beyond, while a third type is not adequately explained by either pathway alone. These paths may be clearly distinguished from the degradation of tryptophan in *E. coli* by tryptophanase or in Neurospora by tryptophan desmolase. The pathways of tryptophan degradation in higher plants appear to be somewhat different from all of these. Shall we assume that the primeval cell possessed all of these routes and evolved to the present biochemical heterogeneity by loss of most of these enzymes?

Carbohydrate metabolism is another area in which an examination of multiple pathways is instructive. In the studies of my laboratory on carbohydrate metabolism in *E. coli,* two major pathways of glucose-6-phosphate metabolism were observed, namely, the phosphogluconate and glycolytic pathways. Both pathways were shown to operate in the growing bacterium. Virus infection affected the balance of these paths and virus appeared to mediate its effects on carbohydrate metabolism by relatively remote disturbances in nucleic-acid metabolism. The appropriate choice of substrate also affected the operation of these systems. In other bacteria, heredity has determined that Leuconostoc mesenteroides shall lack the glycolytic pathway and operate exclusively via phosphogluconate. Conversely, *Lactobacillus casei* uses only the glycolytic pathway in anaerobic and aerobic growth. These pathways are also present in the mammal; recent data indicate that differentiation has concentrated the phosphogluconate path in the liver and the Embden-Meyerhof scheme in muscle. In *B. subtilis,* a diet of amino acids permits the normal operation of both paths. Deprived of exogenous amino acids, *B. subtilis* lacks key enzymes of the Embden-Meyerhof scheme and is constrained by these nutritional conditions to one of the two pathways. Thus, the quantitative significance of these basic systems are determined by heredity, differentiation, nutrition, virus infection, and the carbohydrate substrate offered.

In addition to these systems, an anaerobic cleavage of phosphogluconate to triose phosphate and pyruvate has been observed in strains of *Pseudomonas.* And in *Aerobacter, Pseudomonas,* etc. there is also a nonphosphorylative pathway by which glucose is converted to gluconate, 2- or 5-ketogluconate, 2,5-diketogluconate, etc., a pathway which is not found in the mammal. Thus, it seems reasonable, in view of all these possibilities, to ask how any parasite does metabolize glucose in contrast to the tissue it infects.

It is evident at this point that we may run into quantitative differences rather than clear differences in quality, such as the presence of an essential metabolite in the parasite and its total absence in the host. Nevertheless, even if a given pathway is the same in host and parasite, important differences may be evident in enzymes catalyzing similar reactions.

For example, the glucose dehydrogenase of liver functions with a pyridine nucleotide, DPN or TPN. The same enzyme of molds, e.g., *Penicillium,* uses FAD as coenzyme. Do not such differences suggest the possibility of marked differences in the protein configurations of the enzymes, and hence suggest the possibility of an independent evolutionary origin rather than a transformation of one into the other?

Quite apart from these evolutionary considerations, differences of this type are important in terms of metabolic inhibition and chemotherapy. For example, aldolase is a Fe^{++}-containing enzyme in both yeast and *Clostridium perfringens* and is susceptible to inhibition by various compounds chelating with the metal. In muscle or higher plants, this enzyme lacks the metal and is not inhibited in this fashion.

There are many other questions related to the problem of metabolic difference and a rational chemotherapy. Certainly it is possible to list many more examples of metabolic difference among various cell types than I have herein presented. I do not wish to imply that major metabolic similarities do not exist but rather consider that they are being weighted in such a manner as to obscure the diversity of existing data. I consider that such an emphasis impedes the development of a rational chemotherapy. It seems evident to me that if a biochemist believes that the same metabolic systems are operating in host and parasite alike, he will not hope to be able to select an inhibitor which will affect the parasite alone.

The facts which I have mentioned indicate important biochemical variability in structural and enzymatic constituents of cells and in functioning metabolic systems in various intact organisms. I would interpret this to mean that the hypothesis of a "unity of biochemistry" is as yet unproven, and that a far greater collection and organization of data are necessary to permit a suitable evaluation and perhaps a more careful formulation of the hypothesis. It seems to me that "comparative biochemistry," if properly redefined without built-in assumptions, can become the discipline entrusted with the collection and organization of these data.

I would suggest that the working definition of comparative biochemistry be expanded in the light of its responsibilities in the study of subjects such as biochemical evolution and chemotherapy. Such a definition might state that comparative biochemistry is "the study of the origin, nature, and control of biochemical variability."

INFORMAL DISCUSSION

D. NACHMANSOHN: Not being a microbiologist I would like to comment on two aspects of more general interest.

The notion of the "biochemical unity of life" is not of recent origin, it has been cherished by Pasteur in the last century and was instrumental in the development of modern dynamic biochemistry. This notion implies that fundamentally similar patterns of chemical mechanisms may be found in all living cells. The energy-yielding reactions, for instance, as discussed by H. A. Krebs, show a surprisingly close similarity and only minor deviations. The notion was the guiding principle in Otto Meyerhof's approach to the study of the sequence of energy transformations in the glycolytic cycle and in spite of the difference of the end products of alcoholic fermentation in yeast and glycolysis in muscle, each progress in one field was analyzed for its possible implications in the other. Very few notions were so fruitful for the progress of our knowledge and this in itself is a full justification and shows its great value. Microbiology, in fact, attracted for that very reason the interest of so many biochemists, offering a useful material for the study of enzymic mechanisms of general interest. Unity, however, was never understood to be identity, as the just-mentioned processes of fermentation and glycolysis show. Deviations even in patterns are familiar to every biochemist. Certainly, in regard to proteins we would anticipate differences according to the milieu, interieur and exterieur; body temperature; special requirements of the great variety of species; etc. It is neither a contradiction to the notion of biochemical unity of life, nor indeed surprising to find, as demonstrated by Dr. Bueding, that the enzyme proteins of schistosomes show variations in respect to pH optimum, K_m, or other physicochemical constants.

The second comment which I would like to make concerns a factor which should be considered in chemotherapy in addition to species differences of enzyme characteristics, and that is permeability. This factor has been briefly mentioned by Dr. Davis, but it should perhaps be more stressed. It plays a very important, if not decisive, role in large sections of pharmacology. The most potent drugs acting upon neuromuscular systems act selectively upon very special foci due to permeability barriers protecting the rest of the tissue. This is the basis of their usefulness. Compounds may sometimes readily penetrate microorganisms and inactivate vital enzymes in concentrations harmless to the host. In case of extracellular invasion they may not even enter host cells because the latter are protected by permeability barriers. The great variations of structure and chemical composition of cellular membranes may offer a basis for modifying specific enzyme inhibitors in a way which leads to destruction of invading organisms without harm to the host. Small changes of molecular structure of the drug may, as is well known, change drastically its ability to penetrate into the interior of some cells and not into that of others.

E. RACKER: I would like to second Dr. Nachmansohn's suggestion that we place more emphasis on differences in permeability. It is well known that certain phosphorylated intermediates of carbohydrate metabolism (e.g., fructose-1,6-diphosphate) can be utilized by some microbial cells but do not seem to penetrate readily into animal cells. Thiamine pyrophosphate is quite readily utilized by some pathogens (*N. gonorrhoeae, B. tularense,* and *H. piscium*) but animal tissues are impermeable to this compound. As far as I know no concerted effort has been made to explore this particular differentiating feature of "disunity in permeability" of phosphorylated compounds. Dr. Philip J. Griffin in our laboratory has recently made preliminary attempts in this direction. Glycolaldehyde phosphate, which was used as an analogue of the intermediate glyceraldehyde-3-phosphate, was found to be effective as inhibitor of growth of *N. gonorrhoeae* and *B. proteus*. Phosphorylated analogues of vitamins are now also being investigated.

In regard to the discussion of unity and disunity in biochemistry I think most of us are aware that we are dealing mainly with a problem in semantics. But disunity in language has led to wars before and I have met "disunitarians in biochemistry" who rank the "unitarians" with the teleologists—a group of people one would not want to associate with, though one might consider borrowing money from them.

However, I believe that this discussion is fruitful in the sense that it may shed light on the specific areas in which a search for differences is likely to be profitable. The structural and chemical differences in the cell wall and membrane, which were discussed by Dr. Stanier, may represent a new starting point for the investigation of differences in permeability and appear to me to be a most promising approach to a rational chemotherapy. While on the other hand the patterns and mechanisms of intracellular biochemical reactions in various cells show remarkable similarity, we must still search for the finer variations and per-"mutations," if we wish to recognize the individual trees of the proverbial forest.

H. A. Krebs: Dr. Cohen has challenged the justification of speaking of a "unity" of the biochemical organization of different organisms. I believe there is some misunderstanding. Species are, of course, distinguished by a very large number of biochemical differences, but when speaking of unity we have in mind the fact that the basic components of living matter are shared by different organisms. The situation has been effectively illustrated by a remark made by Albrecht Kossel in 1912 which I would like to quote. But I should first recall that earlier generations of biologists were impressed by the differences between organisms which strike the eye. Immunology had shown qualitative chemical differences even between individuals of the same species. Differences, therefore, were taken for granted when the pioneers of biochemistry discovered the very same amino acids and nucleic acids in all types of living organisms. It is true that special substances are occasionally encountered— like diaminopimelic acid or hydroxymethyl cytosine—which are not shared by all organisms. But the fact remains that many basic substances are common to all organisms. We have reasons for assuming, as I have tried to explain earlier, that the energy-producing mechanisms have also common features in all living matter. In this sense the "unity" of the biochemical organization is a fact which does not require further proof. But if the basic units are shared there is still scope for variety and differences, and I am now coming to Kossel's point. (Kossel, A. (1912). *Johns Hopkins Hosp. Bull.* 23, 65.) He remarked "We obtain some idea of the possible variety in the combinations and reactions of the protein constituents by recalling the fact that they are as numerous as the letters of the alphabet which are capable of expressing an infinite number of thoughts."

Thus unity and variety do not exclude each other. Unity refers merely to some of the basic principles which are employed by living matter. By modifying the basic units and mechanisms and by using different permutations and combinations in the final build-up living matter can achieve a uniqueness of individuals even of the same species.

S. E. Luria: Concerning the unity of biochemistry (insofar as it influences our thinking about infection, host-parasite specificities, and chemotherapy), clearly the basic unity reflects the common information system used by all organisms in building protoplasm—about 20 digits (= amino acids) for proteins, as pointed out by Dr. Krebs, and, even more restrictively, 5 or 6 digits (= nucleotides) for desoxyribonucleic acids. On this common basis, however, the organic world is developing innumerable diversified metabolic instruments and synthesizing elaborate and *specific* patterns of complex molecules. At this level, the main unity-enforcing agency becomes natural selection, which handicaps any configuration deviant enough to impair the efficiency of essential functions. As a consequence, we may expect to find a given metabolic result to be obtained in different organisms either by the same mechanism or by very dissimilar, but (*mutatis mutandis*) equally efficient mechanisms.

E. Bueding: I am in complete agreement with Dr. Stanier and Dr. Cohen who have pointed out that there has been a tendency to overemphasize the uniformity of biochemical reactions to such an extent that biochemical species differences have been overlooked and neglected. In the study of these problems differences and similarities deserve equal attention and a one-sided view is liable to result in a distorted and inadequate concept. Perhaps this point may be illustrated with an analogy from an entirely different field. If, on hearing variations to a musical theme, we were seeking to recognize only the thematic material, but to ignore all other features of the work, we would accumulate a series of disconnected episodes exhibiting similar characteristics; yet, we would be utterly unable to understand or to appreciate the composition as a complex, but unified structure containing both similar and diverse elements.

W. Vishniac: In a discussion of our present-day attitude toward the concept of comparative biochemistry it is, I believe, pertinent to recall some of the points which Kluyver raised in his now famous paper "On the Unity in Biochemistry." (Kluyver, A. J. and Donker, H. J. L. (1926). *Chem. Zelle u. Gewebe* 13, 134.) A good deal has been said today against the naive view of unified biochemistry, the view that the main biochemical features are identical in all organisms. We do not hold such an extreme view today, nor is it fair to impute to Kluyver this oversimplified version of comparative biochemistry. The only sweeping generalization in which Kluyver indulged was his interpretation of biochemical processes as hydrogen transfer reactions. The universal importance of intermediate hydrogen transfer reactions has certainly been borne out by later studies. Our present knowledge of intermediate reactions in various organisms requires a reappraisal of our ideas concerning comparative biochemistry as Dr. Cohen has just pointed out.

I would like to take this opportunity to point out one of the major achievements of comparative biochemistry. For many years the autotrophic bacteria and plants were thought to be entirely distinct physiologically from the heterotrophic microorganisms and animals. Kluyver's ideas contributed greatly to breaking down this artificial barrier and to the recognition of biochemical characters which autotrophs and heterotrophs have in common.

W. W. Umbreit: There is only one point on which I might comment. Dr. Davis points out that when resistance develops to a drug it is unlikely that a new metabolic pathway is established since it is difficult to see how a genetic change, required for resistance, should be able to *add* a metabolic reaction. While one must admit that logic is on the side of Dr. Davis, the studies on streptomycin and resistance to it appear to show otherwise. Streptomycin is a most inconvenient drug from this point of view since not only in its mode of action but also in the resistance pattern it does not appear exactly logical.

Studies on resistant strains show that a wide variety of metabolic patterns may be observed in the resistant strain, but that, whatever else may have happened, the streptomycin-sensitive "oxalacetate-pyruvate" reaction seems to have disappeared. This is the difficulty, of course, since it is almost impossible to be sure that a reaction is completely absent, especially one of this sort, which can only be measured indirectly. But except for this uncertainty, the data demonstrate that the antibiotic-sensitive reaction is missing. This reaction leads to the formation of a seven-carbon phosphorylated intermediate. We have now been able to isolate this substance from the resistant strain grown in the presence of streptomycin. If, therefore, the streptomycin-sensitive reaction is absent (or inhibited due to the presence of streptomycin during growth of the resistant strain) but the product of the reaction has been formed, an alternative route to that product must have been present, whether logical or not.

E. RACKER: Dr. Umbreit, I am not sure I quite followed your reasoning. Does the lack of sensitivity to streptomycin necessarily indicate an alternative route to the formation of the seven-carbon compound, or is it not possible, as Dr. Davis has pointed out, that the enzyme protein has been altered without changing the route? I also wonder whether you would care to tell us more about the chemistry of the seven-carbon compound?

W. W. UMBREIT: It is not the lack of sensitivity to streptomycin which indicates an alternative route, but rather the metabolic studies on the resistant strain in which one is so far unable to find the streptomycin-sensitive type of reaction. It is true that this reaction must be measured indirectly, as was done, for example, by Smith, Oginsky, and Umbreit (1949). *J. Bacteriol.* 58, 761. This reaction is characterized by the complete oxidation to CO_2 and water of a mixture of oxalacetate and pyruvate, and in the sensitive strain with streptomycin the oxidation only to the state of acetate. When the comparable materials were supplied to the resistant strain only oxidation to acetate was observed. At this point one may say that the metabolic studies on resistant strains indicate that the sensitive reaction has been eliminated, although they do not offer absolute and complete proof that it does not exist.

In regard to the seven-carbon compound the essential information which we have about this substance has been published in *J. Bacteriol.* (1953), 66, 74. In essence, this is an acid-stable substance whose barium and mercury salts are insoluble. It would normally occur as a contaminant of ATP or adenylic acid when these are isolated by precipitation methods. The substance is presumed to be 2-phospho-4-hydroxy-4-carboxyadipic acid, based on the characterization of Rapoport and Wagner who first isolated it from dog liver. It proves to be a metabolic intermediate in both animal and bacterial tissue as traced by radioactive phosphorus. Its synthesis in the bacteria occurs only when pyruvate plus a dicarboxy acid (oxalacetate, fumarate, or malate) are present and not when pyruvate alone is supplied, and the synthesis is inhibited by concentrations of streptomycin which are comparable to those required to inhibit growth.

PART II

METABOLIC ASPECTS OF THE INFECTIOUS PROCESS

THE TISSUES AND BODY FLUIDS AS MEDIA FOR PATHOGENIC AGENTS

By René J. Dubos, *The Rockefeller Institute for Medical Research, New York 21, New York*

ALL TEXTBOOKS of infectious diseases dutifully begin with a chapter devoted to metabolic chemistry, but in practice, metabolic knowledge is not used in the analysis of infectious processes. The reason is simply that despite its spectacular advances during the past three decades, the science of microbial metabolism and physiology has contributed but little to the understanding of reactions between host and parasite.

It is often said that the ignorance concerning the biochemical aspects of infection is due to the fact that, with a few exceptions, students of microbial metabolism have used in their studies microorganisms never encountered in disease, and have almost completely neglected pathogenic agents. I doubt the validity of this explanation. Had the biochemists investigated the metabolism of group A hemolytic streptococci, or of anthrax bacilli, or of typhoid bacilli, they would have discovered that these organisms derive energy and carry out organic syntheses by chemical reactions identical with those recognized in lactic acid streptococci, *Bac. megatherium,* or *Escherichia coli.* The genius of metabolic chemistry during our era has been to unravel fundamental processes common to most living things, but it is not in these aspects of metabolism that pathogens differ from saprophytes. Instead, pathogenic behavior seems to depend upon a combination of minor and subtle peculiarities of the infective agents which permit them to survive, multiply, and cause damage in specific *in vivo* environments. And since all animal species, including man, utilize the same fundamental metabolic processes, the determinants of pathogenicity must be sought for in differences so trivial from the point of view of general physiology, that they escape the attention of those concerned with the general biochemical phenomena of life.

As one tries to discover a metabolic basis for pathogenicity. it soon becomes apparent that the first question to be answered is not why pathogens can cause disease, but rather why saprophytes do not proliferate as well as pathogens—or at all—*in vivo*. Tissues and body fluids contain almost every kind of nutrient; they exhibit in different parts of the body a range of oxygen and CO_2 tensions wide enough to provide almost every type of gaseous atmosphere; even H^+ concentrations are found to vary from pH 3.5 to pH 7.5 in various body areas. Since saprophytes are considered as a rule to be less exacting than pathogens in their growth requirements, it seems at first sight very surprising that they fail to establish themselves and multiply in the animal body. The answer to this riddle will certainly be found in one aspect of the problem which is rarely mentioned and never studied, namely the very special types of environment which micro-organisms find in animal tissues.

Much is known of course of the physiological *"milieu interieur"* maintained approximately constant by the homeostatic mechanisms of the body. It must be realized, however, that this *milieu interieur* refers only to the extracellular environment in which blood and tissue cells are bathed under normal conditions, and is not the environment in which the infectious process follows its course. For it is certain that immediately after penetrating the body, microbial agents find themselves under conditions profoundly different from those termed "physiological."

In vivo, most pathogens as well as saprophytes are rapidly engulfed by various types of phagocytic cells. Some immediately become surrounded by a vacuole, others appear to remain free within the cytoplasm. Hardly anything is known of the inorganic, organic, and gaseous environments that prevail within these phagocytic cells, in or out of the vacuoles, and what little is known adds to the complexities of the problem. There are indications, for example, that following engulfment of certain types of foreign particles and microorganisms, the intracellular pH falls to a very low level, at least inside the phagocytic vacuole (9, 11, 13). There is also the important fact that the various types of phagocytic cells differ in some of their chemical activities. Recent findings suggest, furthermore, that cellular metabolism is modified during metabolic disorders (natural diabetes or alloxan diabetes), and can be altered by hormones (6, 7). It is clear, therefore, that understanding of the metabolic aspects of intracellular infections—and these are the cause of by far the largest number of infectious diseases and of the most important ones—will demand a new type of biochemical knowledge of both host and parasitic cells, for which techniques of study have not even been developed yet.

The problem is hardly simpler for extracellular infections. It is true that microorganisms find at first in blood and lymph, conditions not too unlike those commonly used in metabolic studies. But this early "physiological" phase of the infection does not last long. The host responds to the presence of parasites by the complex and variable reactions referred to under the generic name of inflammation, and there is no doubt that the inflammatory zone is far different biochemically from the normal tissues and body fluids. Whatever the nature of the irritant, inanimate material or living parasite, the inflammatory area is the site of intense glycolytic metabolism on the part of inflammatory and perhaps also of fixed tissue cells: glucose is used up, lactic acid accumulates, and the pH is lowered; there is a decrease in oxygen and an increase in CO_2 tension; alterations in the vascular bed bring about changes in its permeability and in blood flow (8, 12). Furthermore, activation of plasma proteases and the autolytic reactions which follow necrosis result in the release of a variety of tissue constituents and breakdown products. All these occurrences are modified qualitatively and quantitatively by the type of infectious agents that bring them forth, by the physiological state of the infected host, and by the particular anatomical location when inflammation occurs (reviewed in reference 2).

It must be kept in mind also that there normally exist in the different tissues and body fluids a host of substances which can under the proper conditions exert toxic effects on microorganisms, and which tend to accumulate, or be activated, in inflammatory and necrotic areas—particularly as a result of reactions associated with immunity and allergy.

The physicochemical characteristics of the tissues markedly influence the survival and multiplication of microorganisms, and have also qualitative effects on their biological properties. Relatively small differences in the physicochemical environment can profoundly influence phenotypic expressions like the production of toxins or the accumulation of surface antigens, as well as heritable characters resulting in marked changes in the microbial populations. In a few cases, some knowledge is available of the metabolic factors which condition the selection of mutants and thus bring about hereditary changes in the microbial population. For example, *Brucella* grown in media in which alanine is allowed to accumulate tend to change from the S to the R colonial type. This change requires the presence of Mn^{++} ions and is inhibited by the presence in the medium of chelating agents which bind this cation (cf. 1). It is also under the control of some serum constituents, the concentration of which varies from one species of animal to another, and with the state of disease or of immunity. Since the S vs. R colonial characteristics in *Brucella* are of significance for pathogenicity, we have here an inkling of the manner in which the biochemical environment can affect the course of the infectious process by modifying the microbial population through hereditary changes in its components.

It is in these subtle complexities of the *in vivo* environment that the explanation of the extraordinary specific character of the phenomena of pathogenicity resides. The pathogenic potentialities of a given microorganism, including its ability to survive and multiply *in vivo* as well as to cause pathological disturbances, can hardly be revealed by studying its behavior in a stereotyped medium selected for the convenience of biochemical analysis. An understanding of pathogenesis demands that the phenomena of growth and of toxicity be observed under the highly specialized environmental characteristics of each host, and of each phase of the infection.

In order to render more apparent the necessity of considering the local tissue environment in the metabolic study of infectious processes, it may be worth while to outline in very broad terms a few special problems which can be apprehended only in the light of this point of view.

Let us examine, for example, the behavior *in vivo* of the strains of viruses or bacteria which are used as living vaccines for immunization against certain virulent infections. In general, the strains of yellow-fever virus (17 D), Newcastle virus (NDV-B), *Myc. tuberculosis* (BCG), *B. anthracis* (Pasteur's first and second vaccine), *B. pestis* (Girard and Otten strains), *Br. abortus* (19), etc., which are used to protect against yellow fever, Newcastle disease, anthrax, tuberculosis, plague, brucellosis, etc., are referred to as "avirulent" because they do not cause fatal disease in experimental animals or man under usual conditions. There is no doubt, however, that these "avirulent" microorganisms do multiply extensively in the tissues and body fluids of the vaccinated hosts; it is for this reason that Pasteur wisely referred to them as "attenuated" in preference to "avirulent." Indeed, it is by virtue of their ability to cause a definite, if abortive, disease that they can elicit immunity against virulent infection. Thus the attenuated ("avirulent") forms used for vaccination differ from the virulent parent strains only quantitatively—by the fact that their proliferation *in vivo* is not extensive or prolonged enough to lead to overt, fatal disease.

In some cases, at least, the difference in outcome of the infections caused by the virulent and attenuated strains of a given microbial agent is determined by the initial rate at which these agents multiply in certain particular organs of the host under consideration. Yet, this does not mean that, intrinsically, the vaccine strain has a longer replication time than the virulent strain. Indeed, it has been shown that both the virulent and the attenuated strains of a given species multiply at the same rate in certain environments. Thus, in the case of the Newcastle disease virus, the virulent and the vaccine strains multiply at the same rate in extraneural tissues of the chicken (blood, lung, rectum, and spleen), but the former multiplies much more rapidly than the latter in the brain and this difference can be recognized very soon after infection. In the chick embryo, both strains multiply equally fast in the cells lining the allantoic sac, but they display marked differences in other organs (4, 5).

Even more striking differences have been recognized between virulent (viscerotropic) and attenuated (neurotropic) strains of yellow-fever virus. If monkeys are inoculated peripherally with a mixture of the two strains, the viscerotropic virus multiplies faster than the neurotropic, whereas the reverse is true if the mixture is injected into the brains of mice (14). It is clear, therefore, that the reasons for the differences in virulence between the vaccine and the virulent strains of the viruses under consideration must be looked for in differences in their response to the normal biochemical environment of certain specific organs.

Quantitative bacteriological experiments with virulent and attenuated (so-called avirulent) BCG strains of tubercle bacilli in the mouse have revealed phenomena of a similar nature (2, 10). However small the dose of BCG bacilli injected, these organisms invade the various organs and proliferate in them. However large the dose, on the other hand, they multiply more slowly than do bacilli of the virulent strains, even when extremely small inocula of the latter are used. Furthermore, marked differences also exist between various strains of BCG. Under ordinary culture conditions *in vitro,* however, there is no detectable difference in rate of multiplication among strains of tubercle bacilli possessing different degrees of virulence.

Many and varied are the tissue agencies which modify the microbial population *in vivo* both qualitatively and quantitatively. In this presentation, I shall limit myself to a brief consideration of the influence of certain metabolites on the fate of tubercle bacilli and staphylococci. *In vitro,* the multiplication of these organisms is markedly or totally inhibited in an environment characterized by the presence of 0.02 M lactic acid, a reaction of pH 6.5, low oxygen tension, and increased CO_2 tension. This type of environment is representative of that created in cellular exudates by vascular thrombosis and by the metabolism of inflammatory cells under normal physiological conditions. But the biochemical response of the body is not always normal. Certain metabolic disturbances probably reflect themselves in the form of peculiarities of the physicochemical environment prevailing in inflammatory areas.

The fact that uncontrolled diabetes and starvation markedly increase susceptibility to several types of microbial diseases led us to undertake a study of the effect on bacterial growth of substances likely to accumulate under conditions of ketosis. It was found that staphylococci and tubercle bacilli (as well as other microbial species) became much more resistant to a variety of inimical situations when lactic acid was replaced in the medium by certain keto acids or polycarboxylic acids. Indeed, the addition of some of these substances to culture media permits many of the bacteria studied to multiply even at very low pH, at reduced oxygen tension, and in the presence of otherwise toxic concentrations of lactic acid (2, 3). In general, the presence of keto and dicarboxylic acids greatly increases the range of conditions under which pathogenic bacteria can grow and survive.

It is not yet possible to relate these *in vitro* findings to the events of infection. Nevertheless, we have begun to institute experiments aimed at developing an experimental approach *in vivo* to the problem of metabolic state and susceptibility to infection. One technique consists in administering thyroid extract or dinitrophenol to mice on an optimal diet in order to increase their metabolism. Another consists in the use of diets designed to induce ketosis, the diet most extensively studied so far being low in protein (6 per cent skim milk), high in glycerides of short-chain fatty acids (20 per cent cocoa butter), and containing 6 per cent sodium citrate.

No convincing biochemical evidence has yet been obtained that mice can be rendered consistently diabetic or acidotic by these treatments. On the other hand, infection tests leave no doubt that administration of thyroid extract, or of dinitrophenol, or of diets that are presumably ketogenic, increases markedly their susceptibility to infection with tubercle bacilli and staphylococci, and even with an attenuated organism like BCG.

Needless to say, these experiments are far too crude to permit a metabolic analysis of the significance of their results. But they show that the course of the infectious process is markedly influenced—indeed, determined—by the physicochemical environment of the tissues. This environment is not that of the body as a whole, but rather the very specialized situation created in each particular lesion by anatomical structure, hormonal control, physiological state, allergic reactions, etc. In this sense, it is possible to speak of a local state of resistance different from the general immunological state of the body, and yet influenced by it. This accounts for the commonly observed fact that the infective agent can thrive and produce progressive disease in one part of an organ while being held in check in another area of the body, and even indeed within the same organ.

In many respects, the problems of medical microbiology demand the kind of conceptual approach that was formulated by S. Winogradski for the study of soil microbiology. Winogradski pointed out the fallacy of attempting to derive conclusions concerning the role of microorganisms in soil processes from the study of their behavior in artificial culture media under conditions designed for the convenience of microbiological and chemical experiments. He advocated the development of new techniques that would permit the study of microbial activities in an environment as similar as possible to that found in the soil.

We need not consider here the obvious difficulties and limitations of this approach when applied to the study of infectious processes. But granted that it is not practically possible to define in chemical terms the continuously changing environment in which infection proceeds, we must recognize nevertheless that no metabolic analysis of microbial disease is possible until an ecological concept is introduced to formulate the problem. It is because this ecological concept has been lacking almost completely heretofore, that bacterial biochemistry has contributed so little to the understanding of pathogenesis.

Winogradski pointed out that each fragment of soil constitutes a biosphere with its own chemical and biological peculiarities. Similarly, the histological study of diseased tissue leaves no doubt that, even within the same organ, there can occur many types of lesions which provide for the infective agent a whole range of metabolic conditions. It would be impossible naturally to provide a complete account—in space and in time—of the biochemical environment during the whole course of each type of infection. But it is possible to study some of the factors which play a part in determining quantitatively and qualitatively the fate of microorganisms *in vivo*, as well as the reaction of tissues to their presence. It is the interplay of these factors which decides whether infection regresses spontaneously or progresses far enough to express itself in overt disease.

REFERENCES

1. Braun, W. (1947). *Bacteriol. Revs.* 11, 75.
2. Dubos, R. J. (1954). Biochemical Determinants of Microbial Diseases. Harvard University Press, Cambridge, Mass.
3. Dubos, R. J. (1953). *J. Exptl. Med.* 98, 145.
4. Karzon, D. T., and Bang, F. B. (1951). *J. Exptl. Med.* 93, 267.
5. Liu, C., and Bang, F. B. (1953). *J. Immunol.* 70, 538.
6. Martin, S. P., Chaudhuri, S. N., Green, R., and McKinney, G. R. (1954). *J. Clin. Invest.* 33, 358.
7. Martin, S. P., McKinney, G. R., Green, R., and Becker, C. (1953). *J. Clin. Invest.* 32, 1171.
8. Menkin, V. (1940). Dynamics of Inflamation. The Macmillan Co., New York.
9. Metchnikoff, E. (1905). Immunity of Infectious Diseases, p. 181. Cambridge University Press, England.
10. Pierce, C. H., Dubos, R. J., and Schaefer, W. B. (1953). *J. Exptl. Med.* 97, 189.
11. Pulcher, C. (1927). *Boll. soc. ital. biol. sper.* 2, 223, 722.
12. Rich, A. R. (1936). *Arch. Pathol.* 22, 228.
13. Rous, P. (1925). *J. Exptl. Med.* 41, 379, 399.
14. Theiler, M. (1951). *in* Yellow Fever, ed. by G. K. Strode, p. 125. McGraw-Hill Book Co., New York.

SOME EFFECTS OF BACTERIA AND THEIR PRODUCTS ON HOST-CELL METABOLISM

By A. M. Pappenheimer, Jr., *Department of Microbiology, New York University College of Medicine*

To cause disease, a microorganism must first penetrate the primary mechanisms of the host's defense. Either it must release a diffusible toxin which is absorbed by the susceptible animal or it must itself gain access to the tissues and multiply therein.

We know a good deal about the armamentaria of certain pathogenic bacteria which enable them to resist and even to destroy the host defenses. Group *A* hemolytic streptococci, for example, may form capsules (hyaluronic acid) and surface components (*M*-proteins) which protect them from phagocytosis. These organisms produce cytotoxins capable of destroying both red and white blood cells. They release the enzyme hyaluronidase—a "spreading factor" which breaks down the intracellular ground substance. Hemolytic streptococci can often cope successfully with one of the host's most potent mechanisms of defense—the inflammatory reaction. By their release of streptokinase, the hosts own plasminogen is activated to form plasmin which dissolves the fibrin barrier; exudates of white cells destroyed by streptococcal cytotoxins are liquefied by streptococcal desoxyribonuclease and the bacteria multiply and continue to spread throughout the tissues.

We likewise know something about the primary protective mechanisms of the host. By means of the inflammatory response the infectious agent is localized; there is a migration of phagocytic cells to the site of invasion and a fibrin barrier is laid down. Within the lesion or inflamed area, under certain conditions tissue breakdown occurs, anaerobic conditions may be set up, and a variety of substances may be produced locally which are inimical for bacteria. Thus, as Dubos has shown (11), Mycobacteria are killed when exposed under anaerobic conditions to traces of organic acids, particularly to lactic acid. Hirsch and Dubos (17) have shown that many tissues contain the enzyme spermine oxidase which oxidizes the base, spermine, also widely distributed in the tissues, to a product which is toxic for Mycobacteria and other organisms. Watson and Bloom (48) and Hirsch and Dubos (18) have extracted from certain animal tissues basic polypeptides of high lysine content, which inhibit bacterial growth.

The host frequently responds to bacterial invasion by a rise in temperature and this must be regarded as a defense mechanism. In some instances, the degree of fever may be sufficient to prevent multiplication or even to kill the invading parasite (13, 23). Finally, if the host withstands the initial onslaught of the invading microorganisms its immune mechanism may be brought into play to neutralize toxins or promote phagocytosis.

This brief introduction serves to provide us with a simplified concept of how, once bacteria have gained access to the body, they may grow, multiply, and spread throughout animal tissues, and of how the host responds to counteract the invasion. It does not provide us with an answer as to how bacteria cause disease and we remain in almost complete ignorance regarding the primary biochemical lesion caused by bacteria growing in the host tissues and of how multiplication of bacteria within the body precipitates a chain of events leading to the symptoms of disease and perhaps to death. It is, of course, obvious that each infectious disease presents its own distinct problem and there are perhaps almost as many mechanisms as there are infectious diseases. The mere fact that the clinician can frequently diagnose correctly the causative organism on the basis of clinical findings alone suggests that the underlying disruption of host-cell metabolism will not be the same for each host-parasite system.

It is our purpose in this chapter to consider some of the possible ways that bacteria or their products may cause biochemical injury to the host cell, and to suggest how a few of the problems might be approached experimentally. Despite our scanty knowledge, a few scattered clues exist which may help to guide us in our speculations. For purposes of the present discussion let us consider the following types of disease-producing organisms:

1. Exotoxin-producing bacteria which grow on mucous membranes or in necrotic tissue where they produce diffusible toxins or toxic enzymes which are the actual agents responsible for the symptoms of the disease. This class of organism cannot multiply in living tissue.

2. Parasites which multiply in the host's tissue fluids, but resist phagocytosis and are incapable of intracellular survival.

3. Organisms which multiply within the host's cells before killing them.

I. DISEASES CAUSED BY EXOTOXIN-PRODUCING BACTERIA

Diphtheria is perhaps the most successfully studied example of this class of disease. In diphtheria, the bacilli are rarely found growing anywhere but in "pseudomembranes," usually located in the throat or nasopharynx. There is no evidence that the organisms can ever multiply in living tissue and all of the characteristic symptoms of the disease are caused by a single reasonably well-characterized diffusible protein-diphtheria toxin.[1]

The diphtheria bacillus is an aerobic organism. When grown in an adequate culture medium with aeration and shaking to prevent the formation of clumps, it produces no toxin and the bacteria themselves contain a high concentration of respiratory pigments. The principle respiratory enzyme and terminal oxidase is cytochrome b_1 (30). When grown under identical conditions except that inorganic iron is the limiting factor, the diphtheria bacillus grows normally and forms no toxin (28) until all of the iron in the medium becomes exhausted. After all the iron has been used up, the bacteria continue growing until their total iron and cytochrome content fall to a level determined by the particular strain used. At the same time, diphtheria toxin and free coproporphyrin are released into the culture supernate in amounts equivalent to the decreased bacterial cytochrome concentration. It has been suggested, on the basis of these quantitative findings, that diphtheria toxin is related to the protein moiety of diphtherial cytochrome b_1 and that the toxin may exert its injurious action by interfering in some way with the normal functioning of the cytochrome system in the affected tissues of the host.

It seems certain that diphtheria toxin cannot cause its effects by *direct* interaction with a cytochrome component since even excessive amounts of toxin added to tissue homogenates or slices fail to inhibit respiration within a reasonable length of time. Moreover, a latent period of many hours follows the injection of toxin into the susceptible animal and during this period no symptoms of any kind are demonstrable despite good evidence that the toxin is rapidly fixed by the tissues. Finally, it would appear that, at the most, a very few molecules of toxin are required to kill a susceptible cell. It has therefore been proposed that the toxin acts by blocking synthesis of one or more components of the cytochrome system.

In attempting to verify this hypothesis experimentally the customary laboratory animals used for assay of diphtheria toxin proved unsatisfactory. When homogenates of tissues from intoxicated guinea pigs, rabbits, and pigeons were tested, no striking changes in cytochrome content could be demonstrated, even using necrotic tissue from animals on the verge of death. The only suggestive finding was a small but consistent decrease in succindehydrogenase-cytochrome b activity, relative to cytochrome oxidase activity in tissues from intoxicated as compared with normal animals. In the light of subsequent experiments it would appear that not

---

[1] The toxin has recently been isolated in crystalline form (Pope and Stevens, 37).

all the cells of the injured tissue are affected simultaneously by the toxin and that those which are affected may disintegrate suddenly and completely. Homogenates from intoxicated tissue may, therefore, consist mainly of particles from the essentially normal cells which still remain.

Far more revealing evidence has come from studies on the effect of diphtheria toxin in a large insect, the cecropio silkworm (31). It has been shown by Williams and his associates (50) that the cytochromes of the cecropia largely disappear at the time of pupation and the beginning of diapause. With the termination of pupal diapause and coincident with the onset of adult development, there is a renewed synthesis of the cytochromes. Cytochrome c is the component that is formed most rapidly at first, and only later in adult development, when the flight muscle of the moth is laid down, are cytochromes b and $a+a_3$ synthesized at their maximum rate.

It has been found that cecropia is highly sensitive to diphtheria toxin at particular stages of its development. Thus, small amounts of toxin cause delayed death during the larval and the developing adult stages of the insect, whereas diapausing pupae survive for many weeks after being injected with large doses of toxin. It is noteworthy that adult development is blocked promptly following injection of toxin, but degenerative changes only become apparent after a prolonged latent period of several days.

Despite the fact that even large doses of diphtheria toxin fail to kill diapausing pupae over a period of weeks, the toxin exerts a selective effect at this stage by causing the complete necrosis and disappearance of striated muscle throughout the insect within 6 to 14 days. The heart, brain, fat body, and certain other organs, however, appear to be completely unaffected. It is significant that the cytochrome oxidase inhibitors, KCN and carbon monoxide under pressure, also fail to kill diapausing pupae but do exert a similar selective effect in causing paralysis of striated muscle. Recent work has shown that two separate and distinct respiratory systems exist side by side in cecropia (32).

1. There are tissues which contain cytochromes $b_5{}^2$ and $a+a_3$ as major components and no detectable cytochrome b or c. This system predominates in most of the tissues during pupal diapause and is the only system present in pupal heart muscle and fat body. Cytochrome b_5 can probably serve as a KCN and CO insensitive terminal oxidase and can

---

[2] Cytochrome b_5 (9, 32) is probably identical with cytochrome e, a pigment which Keilin and Hartree (20) have shown to be widely distributed in nature. It is spectroscopically identical with the cytochrome pigment of rat-liver microsomes studied by Strittmatter and Ball (43).

bring about the oxidation of DPNH as shown in Fig. 1. Tissues containing the b_5 system only respire slowly because of the slow rate of oxidation of reduced b_5 by molecular oxygen; they do not oxidize succinate; they are not poisoned by antimycin A and are *unaffected by diphtheria toxin*.

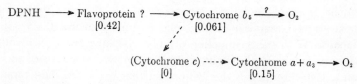

FIG. 1. RESPIRATORY PATHWAY IN DIAPAUSING HEART MUSCLE—TOXIN RESISTANT.
[ ] = activity in micromoles cytochrome c oxidized or reduced per minute per mg N (32).

2. There are tissues which contain cytochromes $a+a_3$, b, and c as major components and cytochrome b_5 as a minor component. This system predominates in striated muscle and particularly in adult flight muscle. This type of tissue oxidizes succinate and reduced coenzyme I (DPNH). Its respiration is sensitive to CO, KCN, antimycin A (38) *and to diphtheria toxin* (see Fig. 2).

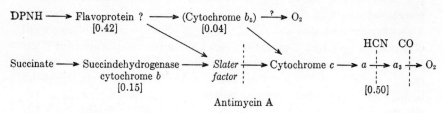

FIG. 2. RESPIRATORY PATHWAY IN DIAPAUSING INTERSEGMENTAL MUSCLE—TOXIN SENSITIVE.
[ ] = activity in micromoles cytochrome c oxidized or reduced per minute per mg N (32).

The experiments with cecropia point strongly to primary involvement of the cytochrome system in the action of the toxin.[3] Moreover, since

[3] There is some evidence which suggests that the chick embryo may vary in susceptibility to diphtheria toxin in a manner analogous to cecropia. It was shown many years ago by Suzuki (45) that tissue cultures from chick embryo are more resistant to diphtheria toxin during the first few days of embryonic development than cultures from later stages. It is of interest that Albaum, Novikoff, and Ogur (2) showed that the succinoxidase activity of chick embryo is low at first and a constant cytochrome oxidase to succinoxidase activity ratio is only reached after the fifth or sixth day of development.

tissues in which cytochromes b_5 and $a+a_3$ predominate are immune to the toxin and since the b_5 and $a+a_3$ contents of intoxicated diapausing pupae are normal (29) we conclude that these components are unlikely to be involved. This leaves cytochromes b, c, and Slater factor as the most likely of the known components to be affected by the toxin. It must be stressed, however, that there is still no evidence for any large decrease of cytochrome b content in intoxicated animals, even cecropia. We have suggested that cytochrome synthesis may be blocked by the toxin and certainly the rapid arrest of adult development in cecropia as compared with the prolonged latent period required before detectable injury occurs to tissue already containing a complete cytochrome system would be in keeping with this hypothesis. However, there are other plausible hypotheses. It is conceivable that diphtheria toxin might alter the arrangement or attachment of the cytochromes in the mitochondria. The toxin might, for example, cause the splitting off of endogenous cytochrome c or might interfere in some way with the coupling of electron transfer and high-energy phosphate-bond formation (Pinchot and Bloom, 34). The absence of a susceptible unicellular organism has rendered elucidation of the mechanism difficult. It would appear that tissue culture technics have not been adequately explored in this connection.

Other bacterial toxins: The modes of action of other bacterial toxins have been studied. There is some indication that the neurotoxin of *Shigella Shiga,* isolated in highly purified form by van Heyningen and Gladstone (46), may also be associated in some way with cytochrome. Shiga neurotoxin is among the most potent of known poisons and its toxicity for the fully susceptible animal, e.g., the rabbit, is equivalent to that of crystalline tetanus (33) or botulinus (1, 22) toxin for the guinea pig, i.e., more than 1000 LD_{50} per microgram toxin per kilo of animal. Like diphtheria toxin, Shiga neurotoxin production is dependent on the iron content of the medium in which the organisms are grown (12, 47). As in the case of the diphtheria bacillus, toxin production and ability to oxidize succinate are inversely proportional, but as van Heyningen and Gladstone (47) have shown, the dysentery bacillus does not form free porphyrin and many more atoms of iron are required to inhibit its formation than are necessary to block diphtheria toxin production.

While the physiological action of the potent neurotoxins produced by *Cl. tetani* and *Cl. botulinum* have been intensively studied since the pioneer work of Marie and Morax (26) and of Meyer and Ransome (27), nothing is known of the primary biochemical injury which these toxins cause to nerve tissue. In the case of botulinus toxin the action would appear to be restricted to the myoneural junctions (5). Recent work by

Burger *et al.* (8) has shown that the neuromuscular block differs from that caused by curare in that nerve conduction is unaffected and the muscle responds normally to direct stimulation. Van Brooks (7) has shown that botulinus toxin interferes with conduction only at the terminal twigs of the motor nerves close to or at the points of final branching and proximal to the site of acetylcholine release.

Finally, mention should be made of the α- or lethal toxin of *Cl. welchii,* one of the causative organisms of gas gangrene. This toxin is an enzyme, a lecithinase which splits lecithin to phosphorylcholine and a diglyceride (24).

II. DISEASES IN WHICH BACTERIA MULTIPLY IN EXTRACELLULAR FLUIDS

In the case of diphtheria we have at least a suggestion as to how the toxin which is responsible for the symptoms of the disease may kill the cells of the host. While it may be a long while before we can furnish final evidence as to the exact mechanism by which toxin interferes with cytochrome in the tissues of the susceptible animal, nonetheless, the theory seems a reasonable one and is corroborated by a considerable body of circumstantial evidence. Let us now enter into speculations regarding another large class of infectious diseases in which the bacteria succeed in gaining entrance to the host tissues and multiply in the extracellular fluids. Pneumococcal lobar pneumonia and anthrax may be considered as typical of this class of disease. Neither the pneumococcus nor the anthrax bacillus produce toxins in artificial culture media which can in any way mimic the symptoms of these diseases when injected into animals.

The lesions in pneumococcal infections and in anthrax are probably due in large measure to the host's response rather than to any specific action of either the bacteria themselves or products released by them. Moreover, enormous numbers (equivalent to many milligrams) of dead bacteria can be injected parenterally into small experimental animals with little demonstrable effect. Equivalent numbers of living avirulent strains can be injected into normal animals or of living virulent organisms into specifically immunized animals with little or no observable effect. By way of contrast, even heat-killed suspensions of many gram negative bacteria such as *E. typhosa* are toxic for laboratory animals. But, in the case of pneumococcus and anthrax bacilli, the mere presence of the bacteria in the body does not suffice to cause disease, and it seems clear that they must not only be present in large numbers but must be actively growing and metabolizing. With some organisms not even active multiplication of large numbers will cause an animal to experience much distress. *Trypanosoma lewisi* and relapsing fever spirochaetes can attain populations in the rat's blood stream which exceed the total number of red blood cells without causing that animal more than the mildest symptoms. In pneumococcal lobar pneumonia in man, pneumococci are found in tremendous numbers in the lungs. Patients who recover from the natural disease without intervention of chemotherapy undergo a dramatic clinical crisis, accompanied by almost complete disappearance of their symptoms, within a matter of a very few hours. The clinical crisis coincides with the appearance of excess antibodies in the blood stream and is attended by a sudden shift of the bacteria into the phagocytic cells where they can no longer multiply and where they are probably killed rapidly. The disappearance of virtually all of the symptoms occurs long before alteration in the gross character of the local lesion has occurred.

What then causes the symptoms in lobar pneumonia if it is neither the lesions in the lungs, nor a specific exotoxin released by the bacteria, nor the mere presence of the organisms in large numbers? How can the metabolism of the bacteria in the tissue fluids interfere with that of the host cells? We can imagine at least two possible mechanisms, neither of which would seem to be beyond experimental approach.

1. There may be competition between bacteria and host cell for an essential metabolite such as a vitamin, an amino acid, or some other growth factor. An organism such as the pneumococcus is probably nearly as fastidious in its nutritive requirements as is the mammalian cell. Pneumococci divide about once every 30 minutes at body temperature and in the face of such rapid multiplication large numbers of pneumococci might conceivably exhaust the local supply of some nutrient within a relatively short time. There seem to be no proven examples of starvation of the host cell caused by growing bacteria during the acute stage of an infectious disease although decreased blood levels of certain growth factors may occur in infected animals. For example, Woodward, Sbarra, and Holtman (51) have demonstrated that infection of white rats with *P. tularensis* results in a marked decrease in the concentrations of some 12 free amino acids in the blood and in the complete disappearance of three of them—cystine, arginine, and phenylalanine. It is conceivable that the rapid bacterial multiplication in tularemia results in depletion of the available free amino acids which in turn causes damage to the host cells by starving them. However, a more likely explanation has been proposed by the authors; namely, that the low free amino-acid concentrations observed may be secondary to severe derangement of metabolism in the liver where the organisms are largely localized. This possibility receives support from their observation that amino-acid levels in recovered rats do not return to normal for some 25 days after infection.

Some interesting examples of competition for growth factors between bacteria and host, in which it is the *host* that is favored, have recently been studied. Thus it has been shown that purine-requiring strains of *E. typhosa* (3) and *Klebsiella pneumoniae* (14) are avirulent for mice when injected intraperitoneally, because mouse peritoneal fluid contains insufficient purine to support their growth. The same strains cause fatal infection if the animals are simultaneously injected with adenine.

2. Bacteria multiplying in the tissue spaces may produce antimetabolites which interfere with some essential step in host cell metabolism, either by competitive inhibition or by some other mechanism. Many examples of microorganisms which produce substances antagonistic to other microorganisms are known and this fact has, of course, led to the isolation of many antibiotics. A considerable proportion of these antagonists have proved toxic for animal tissues. There is no reason why pathogenic bacteria should not produce similar "antibiotics" *in vivo*. This type of diffusible toxin need not be fixed by host cells as are the classical bacterial exotoxins, but would be maintained at effective local concentrations in those tissues where the bacteria are rapidly multiplying. In at least two infectious diseases of plants such a mechanism appears to operate.

The phytopathogenic fungus, *Fusarium lycopersici,* causes a disease of tomato plants in which the leaves curl up and wilt. Both in the infected plant and in artificial culture media the fungus produces a diffusible, low-molecular-weight toxin capable of causing excised tomato leaves to curl and wilt as in the diseased plant. The toxic principle, *lycomarasmin,* was isolated by the Swiss chemists Plattner and Clauson-Kaas (35) who showed it to be a peptide which yielded glycine and aspartic acid upon hydrolysis (36). Woolley (53) has proposed that *lycomarasmin* is a tripeptide composed of asparagine, glycine, and a new amino acid, alpha-hydroxyalanine:

$$\underset{\text{Lycomarasmin}}{\overset{\displaystyle \text{H}_2\text{NOC}-\text{CH}_2 \qquad\qquad\qquad\qquad \text{CH}_3}{\underset{\displaystyle \text{HOOC}-\text{CH}-\text{NH}-\text{CO}-\text{CH}_2-\text{NH}-\text{C}-\text{OH}}{\qquad\qquad\qquad\qquad\qquad\qquad\qquad\qquad \text{COOH}}}}$$

A synthetic peptide of similar structure but differing from the natural peptide in its solubility possessed the same biological activity as lycomarasmin itself (53). Woolley has shown that lycomarasmin antagonizes the growth-promoting activity for bacteria of *strepogenin,* an essential glutamic-acid-containing peptide (52), and that *strepogenin* can relieve, noncompetitively, the toxic effects of small amounts of lycomarasmin in excised tomato-plant leaves.

Recent studies on another plant disease furnish an even more striking and clear-cut example of the pathogenic effect of an antimetabolite produced by an infecting microorganism *in vivo*. The causal agent of wildfire disease of tobacco is a bacterium, *Pseudomonas tabaci*. Braun (6) showed that typical lesions of the disease could be reproduced by a low-molecular-weight toxin elaborated by the pseudomonas grown in artificial culture. Braun further showed that the factor was toxic for the unicellular plant *Chlorella vulgaris* and that its toxicity for chlorella could be specifically and competitively relieved by *l*-methionine but by no other amino acid or growth factor of a large series which he tested. Since precursors of methionine such as homocysteine failed to inhibit the toxicity of the *Pseudomonas* factor, Braun concluded that it is the utilization rather than the synthesis of methionine that is blocked in the disease. Moreover, typical lesions were produced in tobacco-plant leaves by a synthetic antagonist for methionine, methionine sulfoximine. Woolley, Schaffner, and Braun (54) have recently isolated *Pseudomonas tabaci* toxin and have shown it to be a derivative of a new amino acid, α,ε-diamino-β-hydroxypimelic acid, the formula of which is shown below:

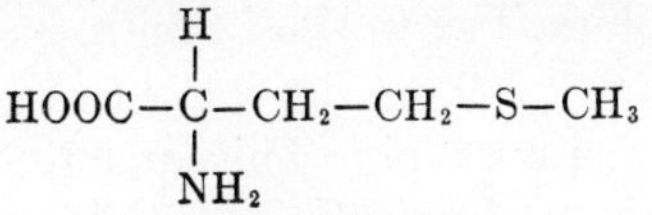

$$\underset{\underset{NH_2}{|}}{HOOC-\overset{\overset{H}{|}}{C}-CH_2-CH_2-S-CH_3}$$

Methionine

$$\underset{\underset{NH_2}{|}}{HOOC-\overset{\overset{H}{|}}{C}-CH_2-CH_2-\overset{\overset{O}{\|}}{\underset{\underset{NH}{\|}}{S}}-CH_3}$$

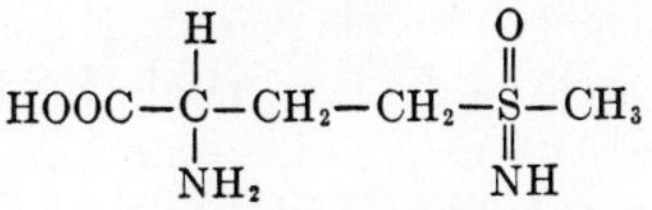

Methionine sulfoxamine

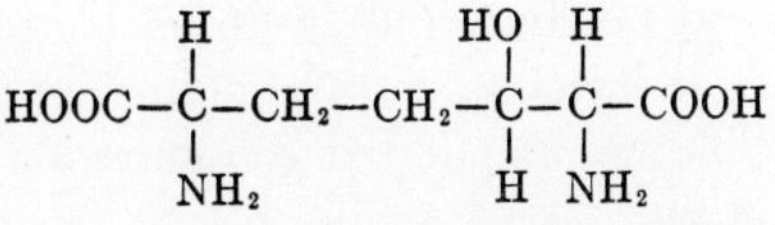

$$\underset{\underset{NH_2}{|}}{HOOC-\overset{\overset{H}{|}}{C}-CH_2-CH_2-\overset{\overset{HO}{|}}{\underset{\underset{H}{|}}{C}}-\overset{\overset{H}{|}}{\underset{\underset{NH_2}{|}}{C}}-COOH}$$

α,ε-diamino-β-hydroxypimelic acid

At least one example of an animal infection can be cited in which the production of an antibiotic by the growing bacteria would appear to be responsible for the local injury observed. *Pseudomonas pyocyanea* is a frequent contaminant of burns and the dressings from such infected burns are often blue-green in color due to the antibiotic pigment, *pyocyanin*, released by the bacteria. Jackson, Lowbury, and Topley (19) have shown that burns infected with the Pseudomonas frequently fail to take skin grafts and that healing is often delayed. Recently, Cruikshank and Lowbury (10) have found that concentrations of only 8 to 24 µg/ml of pure pyocyanin inhibit or kill tissue culture explants of human skin and are toxic for leucocytes. They have extracted pyocyanin from the exudates of burns and found concentrations of the pigment ranging from 8 to over 300 µg/gm of exudate. Such concentrations are well above those which proved to be toxic for leucocytes and for human skin *in vitro*. They point out that the local supply of pyocyanin on the surface of burns is constantly being maintained and replenished by growth of *Pseudomonas pyocyanea*. While Cruikshank and Lowbury's findings with respect to the role of pyocyanin in infected surface lesions appear to be clear-cut, they were unable to demonstrate that pyocyanin was responsible for local lesions produced by intradermal injection of Pseudomonas cultures into laboratory animals.

A mechanism analogous to that which Braun and Woolley have demonstrated in wildfire disease of tobacco might well explain the pathogenesis of bacterial infections such as those caused by the anthrax bacillus or by pneumococci. Moreover, the design of experiments to demonstrate the operation of similar mechanisms in animal infections should not present insurmountable difficulties. The work of Smith, Keppie, and Stanley (41) shows that a minimum of 200 mg dry weight of growing anthrax bacilli are required to kill a guinea pig. This quantity of growing bacterial protoplasm might easily produce sufficient inhibitor in the tissues to reach local concentrations high enough to interfere with host-cell metabolism. Such low-molecular-weight diffusible poisons, if they are not fixed by cells or if they are metabolized by the host, might be difficult to demonstrate by injection of culture filtrates and would presumably be dispersed, diluted, excreted, or metabolized with great rapidity once the bacteria ceased multiplying in the tissues. In the experiments with pyocyanin cited above, Cruikshank and Lowbury (10) were unable to produce lesions in animals by intradermal injection of pyocyanin, presumably because this toxin is freely diffusible and an effective concentration could not be maintained at the injection site.

III. INTRACELLULAR PARASITES

While pneumococci and *B. anthracis* can multiply in great numbers in the extracellular fluids of susceptible animals, the available evidence indicates that once they become engulfed by phagocytic cells they no longer multiply and presumably their survival within the cell is short. There are, however, a number of pathogenic bacteria which probably cause most of their injurious effects by intracellular growth and multiplication. In fact, the malaria parasites, the leprosy bacillus, and the Rickettsia have never been cultivated extracellularly and even in the actual disease itself it would appear that growth only occurs within the cells. In the case of such "obligate" intracellular parasitism the possibility of competition between host cell and invading organism for an essential growth factor should be seriously considered. Indeed, one might venture to speculate that inability of these organisms to grow outside the cell perhaps depends on a requirement for one or more of the less stable, but essential, transient intermediary metabolites which do not exist outside the living cell. Studies on the respiration of the rat leprosy bacillus, *M. lepraemurium,* obtained from infected rat testicles and freed from host tissue components show a fairly high endogenous metabolism [$Q_{o_2} = 40$ to 70 µl/mg N, Gray (16)], despite their extremely slow growth rate. Gray has recently tested over 50 substrates and cofactors including sugars, certain glycolytic intermediates, amino acids, fatty acids, coenzymes, and vitamins without finding a single one capable of stimulating respiration. It is difficult to escape the conclusion that *M. lepraemurium* is impermeable to most of the common substrates. Nevertheless, it is probably not impermeable to all of them since Gray has found that respiration can be stimulated 35 to 50% in the presence of rather high concentrations of yeast or liver extract. In leprosy as well as in other instances of intracellular parasitism, the host cells often survive until literally filled with infecting microorganisms. Perhaps only when their numbers are great do they succeed in bringing about death and lysis of the host cell by exhaustion of an essential metabolite, and so are finally released to be taken up by a fresh host cell.

Suspensions of leucocytes and monocytes rapidly ingest large numbers of many strains of living pathogenic bacteria such as typhoid bacilli, Gram-negative cocci, and both virulent and avirulent tubercle bacilli. Although these phagocytic cells do not actually multiply in so-called "tissue cultures," under suitable conditions they will remain viable for several weeks (Mackaness, 25). The experiments of Suter (44) and of Mackaness (25) show that while both virulent and avirulent tubercle bacilli are taken up by such cell suspensions, it is only the virulent organisms that multiply in and are toxic for the monocytes. The metabolism of such cells before and after ingestion of living virulent or avirulent bacteria does not appear to have received much study. It is to be anticipated that investigations of the metabolism of parasitized cells might well throw a good deal of light on the nature of the primary biochemical damage caused by pathogenic bacteria to the host cell.

IV. CONCLUDING REMARKS

In considering possible mechanisms of biochemical injury to host cells by disease-producing bacteria we have intentionally chosen examples which appeared the simplest and have avoided discussing even those complications we are well aware of. It is certain that we have oversimplified and that because of the enormous number of variables involved the infectious process is often extremely complex. For example, since the time of Bail (4) there have been repeated demonstrations that the anthrax bacillus produces antigens ("aggressins") *in vivo* which under the usual conditions are not found *in vitro* (15, 42, 49).[4] In other words, the parasite can "adapt" itself to the host, and presumably the formation of certain enzymes are induced *in vivo* which play a role in pathogenesis. At least in the case of anthrax it is likely that the adaptation involved is concerned with protection of the bacteria from host defense mechanisms, thereby allowing them to multiply unhindered. Bail's "aggressin" is probably not the factor which causes tissue damage. A further interesting difference between anthrax bacilli grown *in vivo* as opposed to organisms grown in broth is the relative ease with which the bacteria from exudates undergo lysis when suspended in dilute ammonium carbonate (21). A similar example of adaptation to conditions in the host is apparent in the staining properties of certain pathogenic acid-fast bacteria growing *in vivo*. Thus tubercle bacilli from lesions in the animal take up the fat stain, Sudan-Black, whereas the same organisms grown on artificial culture media fail to take up the dye (40).

We have classified invading bacteria according to whether they multiply extracellularly or intracellularly. Many bacteria such as *E. typhosa* and *M. tuberculosis* unquestionably are capable of growth both in the cells and outside them. In the former case, owing to a toxic surface component, it still seems uncertain whether in intracellular growth, the host cells remain living or are killed before growth takes place. In contrast to the pneumococcus, meningococci and typhoid bacilli themselves are toxic for the host and the numbers of heat-killed bacteria required to kill laboratory animals do not appear to differ substantially from the numbers of living bacteria required to cause death following infection. However, in experimental as well as in natural disease, the local site of bacterial multiplication is often of great importance. Thus the experiments of Reilly and his associates (39) have demonstrated that far fewer *S.*

[4] Gladstone (15) succeeded in producing aggressin "*in vitro.*" Two factors are required, one of which is the bicarbonate ion and the other an unidentified factor associated with a protein fraction of blood plasma.

paratyphi B are required to produce fatal infections in laboratory animals when the organisms are introduced directly into the mesenteric lymph nodes than if injected by any other route.

In discussing pneumococcal lobar pneumonia and anthrax it was mentioned that the gross lesions observed in those diseases may be caused by the hosts own nonspecific inflammatory response to the presence of the bacteria. It seems possible that in many chronic infections such as tuberculosis and perhaps even rheumatic fever, the abnormal metabolism of the host may be attributed in large measure to a heightened or exaggerated inflammatory response caused by hypersensitization to the bacteria or to their products. Under these conditions we need no longer search for a primary biochemical injury to the host caused by the *metabolic activity* of the growing infectious agent, and the mere presence of the organisms themselves or their products may suffice to account for all or most of the signs of the disease.

Since the days of Paul Ehrlich, students of infectious disease have sought to find what Sir Paul Fildes has called "a rational approach to chemotherapy." Both by accident and by design, but never by a rational approach, many drugs have been discovered and virtually all bacterial and rickettsial diseases can now be treated successfully by one or another chemotherapeutic agent. During the past few years, our knowledge of the intermediary metabolism of bacteria and of mammalian tissues has advanced rapidly. It may some day become possible to chart the sequence of untoward biochemical events, initiated by an invading microorganism, which lead ultimately to the appearance of disease in the host. Perhaps only when we understand how the metabolism of a pathogenic organism can interfere with the metabolism of the cells of its host will it at last become possible to discover a new chemotherapeutic agent by means of a rational approach.

REFERENCES

1. Abrams, A., Kegeles, G., and Hottle, G. A. (1946). *J. Biol. Chem.* 164, 63.
2. Albaum, H. G., Novikoff, A. B., and Ogur, M. (1946). *J. Biol. Chem.* 165, 125.
3. Bacon, G. A., Burrows, T. W., and Yates, M. (1951). *Brit. J. Exptl. Pathol.* 32, 85.
4. Bail, O. (1904). *Zentr. Bakteriol. Parasitenk. Abt. I* 36, 266.
5. Bishop, G. H. and Bronfenbrenner, J. J. (1936). *Am. J. Physiol.* 117, 393.
6. Braun, A. C. (1950). *Proc. Natl. Acad. Sci. U.S.* 36, 423.
7. Brooks, V. B. (1953). *Science* 117, 334.
8. Burger, A. S., Dickens, F., and Zatman, I. J. (1949). *J. Physiol.* 109, 10.
9. Chance, B. and Pappenheimer, A. M., Jr. (1954). *J. Biol. Chem.* In press.
10. Cruickshank, C. N. D. and Lowbury, E. J. L. (1953). *Brit. J. Exptl. Pathol.* 34, 583.
11. Dubos, R. J. (1953). *J. Exptl. Med.* 97, 357.
12. Dubos, R. J. and Geiger, J. W. (1946). *J. Exptl. Med.* 84, 143.

13. Enders, J. F. and Shaffer, M. F. (1936). *J. Exptl. Med.* 64, 7.
14. Garber, E. D., Hackett, A. J., and Franklin, R. (1952). *Proc. Natl. Acad. Sci. U.S.* 38, 693.
15. Gladstone, G. P. (1946). *Brit. J. Exptl. Pathol.* 27, 394.
16. Gray, C. T. (1952). *J. Bacteriol.* 64, 305.
17. Hirsch, J. G. and Dubos, R. J. (1952). *J. Exptl. Med.* 95, 191; Hirsch, J. G. (1953), *J. Exptl. Med.* 97, 345
18. Hirsch, J. G. and Dubos, R. J. (1954). *J. Exptl. Med.* 99, 65.
19. Jackson, D. M., Lowbury, E. J. L., and Topley, E. (1951). *Lancet* ii, 137.
20. Keilin, D. and Hartree, E. F. (1949). *Nature* 164, 254.
21. Keppie, J., Smith, H., and Harris-Smith, P. W. (1953). *Brit. J. Exptl. Pathol.* 34, 486.
22. Lamanna, C., Eklund, H. W., and McElroy, O. E. (1946). *Science* 103, 613.
23. MacCallum, P., Tolhurst, J. C., Buckle, G., and Sissons, H. A. (1948). *J. Pathol. Bacteriol.* 60, 93.
24. MacFarlane, M. G. and Knight, B. C. J. G. (1941). *Biochem. J.* 35, 884.
25. Mackanness, G. B. (1952). *J. Pathol. Bacteriol.* 64, 429.
26. Marie, A. and Morax, V. (1902). *Ann. inst. Pasteur* 16, 818.
27. Meyer, H. and Ransome, F. (1903). *Arch. Pathol. Pharmacol.* 49, 369.
28. Mitsuhashi, S., Kurokawa, M., and Kojima, Y. (1949). *Japan. J. Exptl. Med.* 20, 261.
29. Pappenheimer, A. M., Jr. Unpublished.
30. Pappenheimer, A. M., Jr. and Hendee, E. D. (1947). *J. Biol. Chem.* 171, 701.
31. Pappenheimer, A. M., Jr. and Williams, C. M. (1952). *J. Gen. Physiol.* 35, 727.
32. Pappenheimer, A. M., Jr. and Williams, C. M. (1954). *J. Biol. Chem.* In press.
33. Pillemer, L., Witler, R. G., and Grossberg, D. B. (1946). *Science* 103, 615.
34. Pinchot, G. B. and Bloom, W. L. (1950). *J. Biol. Chem.* 184, 9.
35. Plattner, P. A. and Clauson-Kaas, N. (1944). *Helv. Chim. Acta* 28, 188.
36. Plattner, P. A. and Clauson-Kaas, N. (1945). *Experientia* 1, 195.
37. Pope, C. G. and Stevens, M. F. (1953). *Lancet* ii, 1190.
38. Potter, V. R. and Reif, A. H. (1952). *J. Biol. Chem.* 194, 287.
39. Reilly, J., Rivalier, E., Compagnon, A., Laplane, R., and duBuit, H. (1935). *Ann. Méd.* 37, 241.
40. Sheenan, H. L. and Whitwell, F. (1949). *J. Pathol. Bacteriol.* 61, 269.
41. Smith, H., Keppie, J., and Stanley, J. L. (1953). *Brit. J. Exptl. Pathol.* 34, 471.
42. Staub, A. M. and Grabar, P. (1944). *Ann. inst. Pasteur* 70, 15.
43. Strittmatter, C. and Ball, E. (1952). *Proc. Natl. Acad. Sci.* 38, 10.
44. Suter, E. (1952). *J. Exptl. Med.* 96, 137.
45. Suzuki, Y. (1918). *J. Immunol.* 3, 233.
46. Van Heyningen, W. E. and Gladstone, G. P. (1952). *Brit. J. Exptl. Pathol.* 34, 202.
47. Van Heyningen, W. E. and Gladstone, G. P. (1952). *Brit. J. Exptl. Pathol.* 34, 221.
48. Watson, D. W. and Bloom, W. L. (1952). *Proc. Soc. Exptl. Biol. Med.* 81, 29.
49. Watson, D. W., Cromartie, W. J., Bloom, W. L., Kegeles, G., and Heckly, R. J. (1946). *J. Infectious Diseases* 80, 1.
50. Williams, C. M. (1948). *Growth* 12, 61.
51. Woodward, J. M., Sbarra, A. J., and Holtman, D. F. (1954). *J. Bacteriol.* 67, 58.
52. Woolley, D. W. (1948). *J. Biol. Chem.* 172, 71.
53. Woolley, D. W. (1948). *J. Biol. Chem.* 176, 1291.
54. Woolley, D. W., Schaffner, G., and Braun, A. C. (1952). *J. Biol. Chem.* 198, 807.

THE ROLE OF HOST POLYSACCHARIDES IN VIRUS REPRODUCTION

By Mark H. Adams, *Department of Microbiology, New York University College of Medicine*

I. INTRODUCTION

Viruses are obligate intracellular parasites, yet in order to survive as living organisms they must be capable of transfer from one host to another. Some viruses are transmitted from generation to generation as if part of the genetic material of the host cell, without the necessity of an extracellular phase; for example, the bacteriophages in lysogenic bacteria. Other viruses are transmitted from host to host only by means of an extracellular phase. This extracellular or "mature" state of the virus must be stable enough to survive outside the host cell during transfer periods and must have some mechanism for attachment to a suitable host cell and for penetration into that cell. In contrast, the intracellular or "vegetative" state of the virus must be capable of survival and reproduction within the host cell. It is already evident that in some cases the vegetative state of a virus is very different in its properties from the mature state. It is a general observation, for instance, that vegetative virus is noninfectious, that is, not transmissable from host to host during the "eclipse" period in the growth cycle of viruses.

I am going to discuss the transition from mature, extracellular virus to vegetative, intracellular virus and the role of host-cell polysaccharides in this change. For examples I will use two of the best known viruses, bacteriophage T2 and its close relatives, and the influenza-mumps group of viruses. There are many other virus systems about which some information is available, and which would contribute to the discussion, but limited space precludes an extensive treatment of this subject.

II. BACTERIOPHAGE

Phage T2 in conventional electron micrographs is sperm shaped with an elliptical head and a short, stout tail. Chemically it consists of a protein membrane and a nucleic-acid core, the nucleic acid being separable from the protein by suitable manipulations. The tail is the organ of attachment, the tail tip becoming fixed to the host-cell surface (4). After adsorption the phage nucleic acid passes into the host cell, leaving the protein membrane on the host-cell surface. The phage protein is a micro-syringe serving to inject the phage nucleic acid, after which the phage protein plays no further role in the infectious process (28). The mature state of T2 phage differs from the vegetative state structurally and chemically as well as physiologically.

Phage Adsorption

The adsorption of phage T2 to its host cell is a very rapid and highly efficient process, the rate-limiting factor being the diffusion of the phage (53). This means that nearly every collision between phage and host-cell surface must result in attachment, and that the bacterial surface is uniform with respect to ability to adsorb this phage. The latter conclusion is substantiated by electron micrographs which show the phage particles randomly distributed over the bacterial surface. Phage adsorption is, however, a highly specific process. The host cell can lose its ability to adsorb the phage particle by a single mutational step, becoming completely phage resistant. The phage in turn can acquire the ability to attack the altered host cell by a mutation which extends its host range (43). The specificity of phage attachment is under the genetic control of both host cell and phage.

That the ionic environment plays a crucial role in the adsorption of phage T2 to its host cell was demonstrated by Hershey, Kalmanson, and Bronfenbrenner (29). The requirement of an organic cofactor such as tryptophane for the closely related phage T4 was discovered by Anderson (2, 3). These environmental requirements for phage adsorption were explained by the work of Puck and collaborators (50, 51). The primary attachment between phage and host cell is electrostatic and readily reversible. Because both phage and host cell have net negative charges, attachment does not occur until some of these charges are neutralized by cations in the environment. The tryptophane plays a similar but more specific role in adjusting the surface-charge distribution on the phage tail. Under appropriate environmental conditions complementary patterns of charge distribution occur on the host-cell surface and the phage tail, ensuring that nearly every approach of phage to bacterium results in adsorption. The effect of pH and chemical reagents on the adsorption of phage T2 to host cells indicates that ionized carboxyl groups of the host cell and ionized amino groups of the T2 phage particle are involved in attachment (58). Experiments on host cell receptors by Weidel (62, 63) are consistent with this view.

Effect of Bacteria on Adsorbed Phage

Under appropriate conditions of ionic environment and temperature, the initial reversible attachment is followed by a second irreversible step. In the case of phage T2 this irreversible step involves release of nucleic acid from the phage particle. Depending on conditions, the phage nucleic acid may enter the host cell and become established there as the vegetative state, or it may be released into the medium with no damage to the host cell (49). A completely satisfactory analysis of the factors which control the decision between these alternatives is not yet available. The release of phage nucleic acid into the medium is undoubtedly responsible for some cases of "abortive infection" (1). Release of phage DNA into the medium also occurs following adsorption of phage T2 to heat-killed bacteria (24) and to fragments of bacterial membranes (28). A highly purified lipocarbohydrate isolated from the host cell is able to inactivate T4 phage, the inactivation being accompanied by release of phage nucleic acid into the medium (39). The ultimate in this direction was the demonstration by Puck and Sagik (50) that the adsorption of phage T2 to a cation-exchange resin results in the release of phage nucleic acid from its protein membrane. Presumably the distribution of sulfonic-acid residues on the resin simulates the pattern of carboxyl residues on the bacterial surface, and is complementary to the charge distribution on the phage particle. Apparently contact of phage T2 with an appropriate configuration of negative charges is enough to stimulate release of the phage nucleic acid. It should be noted that not all phages behave in this way. Phage T1 does not liberate its nucleic acid so readily (50), whereas the nucleic acid is liberated from phage T5 whenever the concentration of cations in the medium is decreased below critical values (41). The destruction of phage T5 has a high energy of activation suggestive of protein denaturation. The energy of activation for the release of T2 or T4 nucleic acid, following contact with suitable surfaces, has not been measured.

Effect of Adsorbed Phage on Bacteria

Adsorbed phage particles may exert a powerful effect on the host cell which is independent of the establishment of infection. Such an effect is "lysis from without" (LFW), which is a prompt lysis of the host cell before the end of the usual latent period and without production of viable phage progeny (13). Lysis from without occurs when 50 to 200 phage particles are adsorbed per bacterium (59), or at much lower multiplicities when metabolic poisons such as cyanide or iodoacetate (11) or dinitrophenol (25) are used. Under appropriate conditions anaerobiosis (11), starvation (25), or ultraviolet irradiation of the bacteria before infection (2, 3) have the same effect as the poisons. Lack of a fermentable energy source (45) also has the same result. These various observations are alike in suggesting that interference with the energy metabolism of the bacterium facilitates LFW.

Phage particles killed by ultraviolet or sonic vibration (2, 3) or X-ray (60) are even more effective than viable T2 phage in causing LFW. Phage T2 membranes produced by osmotic shock and essentially free of nucleic acid are able to cause LFW (27), demonstrating that LFW is independent of the injection of phage nucleic acid into the host cell. Similarly the destruction of bacterial cell membranes by phage suggests that lysis from without is independent of the cytoplasmic constituents of the bacterial cell (61).

Although LFW has been an extremely useful tool in phage research for the premature lysis of infected bacteria (14), there have been few systematic studies of the phenomenon and these few have been contradictory. Weidel (62) has reported the following observations on the effect of phage T2 on host bacteria:

1. Phage T2 disrupts by LFW not only living bacteria but bacteria killed by dilute NaOH, formalin, or heat.

2. A freshly prepared lysate of host bacteria, made by LFW with phage T2, neither kills nor lyses fresh bacteria when these are added. He concluded from these experiments that LFW does not involve the activation of autolytic bacterial enzymes by phage T2, but rather that phage T2 is capable of a direct chemical attack on the bacterial membrane. There is no evidence to date suggesting that phage T2 can be eluted after damaging the bacterial cell membrane, so it is not analogous to the influenza, mumps group of animal viruses.

In direct conflict are the observations and conclusions of Puck (49) on the same phage-host cell system:

1. LFW occurs only under environmental conditions in which irreversible adsorption occurs.

2. In 0.1 M NaCl solution LFW does not occur with single infection but occurs rapidly at a multiplicity of four phage particles per bacterium.

3. LFW is suppressed at 0°C or in 2% phenol, suggesting that an enzymatic process is involved.

4. When virus or host cells are heated to 60°C for 30 min, viable phage plus heated bacteria gave no LFW; heated phage plus viable bacteria gave rapid LFW.

Puck concluded from these observations that phage T2 activates some autolytic bacterial enzyme which is then responsible for cell lysis. Both Puck and Weidel concluded that the lysis is enzymatic but they were diametrically opposed as to the location of the enzyme, whether in the host cell or in the phage particle. There are flaws in the experiments of both authors and only further and more critical experiments can settle this question as to the mechanism of lysis from without. The importance of this question is that LFW may be intimately related to the problem of penetration of phage nucleic acid into the host cell. In this connection it should be noted that not all phages are able to bring about LFW and even in the case of the T2 serological group, the r^+ phages are much more active than the r mutants (25).

Chemical Nature of the Host Receptor Site

It was recognized early that susceptibility of enteric bacteria to some bacteriophage strains was correlated with the possession of certain bacterial antigens (7), hence the terms "Vi" phages and "O" phages. Because the specificity of adsorption was correlated with possession of certain antigens, and the antigenic specificity was due to polysaccharides, it was assumed that the receptor sites must consist of polysaccharides. When purified bacterial polysaccharides were tested for phage neutralizing activity they were usually found to be inert. In contrast crude extracts of host bacteria were very potent phage inhibitors, attempts at purification resulting in decreased activity (10). Such studies led Burnet to the following conclusion (10): "The first stage in the lysis of susceptible bacteria requires the mutual specific union of certain elements of complementary molecular configuration on the surfaces of the phage particle and bacterium respectively. The specific element on the bacterial surface is intimately related to the polysaccharide hapten which determines the antigenic character of the bacterium. The hapten, as finally isolated by chemical methods, is not present as such in the bacterial surface, but forms an essential part of a more complex molecular pattern. It is to certain aspects of this pattern, not necessarily the same for each phage lysing the organism, that specific phage adsorption occurs." More recent work has served only to confirm and to clarify details of this remarkable statement.

More specific information about the chemical nature of bacterial receptors has not come from attempted isolation of the receptor substances but rather as a byproduct of a long-term study of bacterial antigens. Earlier work by Boivin (5) and by Morgan (46) had demonstrated that the "O" antigens of the enteric pathogens consisted of a complex association of polysaccharide, lipid, and protein. Extensive studies of such antigens from various species of *Shigella* have been made by Goebel and collaborators.

The antigen of phase II *Sh. sonnei* was extracted from phenol-killed organisms with warm water and purified by alcohol fractionation. This electrophoretically homogeneous complex of lipocarbohydrate and protein neutralized phages T2, T3, T4, T6, and T7. Digestion with pancreatin, which removed most of the protein, increased its serological and phage-neutralizing activity. Extraction with phenol which removed all detectable protein also destroyed its ability to neutralize phages T2 and T6. The residual lipocarbohydrate, which still neutralized phages T3, T4, and T7, yielded on hydrolysis 45% reducing sugar, 29% lipid, 4% acetyl, 4% phosphorus, and 13% ash. The carbohydrate portion contained glucose, galactose, glucosamine, and a heptose (38). *E. coli* strain B contains a serologically related antigen which has not yet been investigated chemically (20). The tryptophane-requiring strain of phage T4 is neutralized by the phase II *Sh. sonnei* antigen only when tryptophane is present (44).

The mechanism by which the lipocarbohydrate neutralizes the infectivity of phage T4 was studied by Jesaitis and Goebel (39). When a concentrated suspension of phage T4 was permitted to react with the lipocarbohydrate of *Sh. sonnei,* there was a rapid increase in viscosity which paralleled the loss of phage activity. Electron microscopy of the mixture revealed phage ghosts and a tangled mass of filaments 50 to 100 Å in diameter. The subsequent addition of desoxyribonuclease caused a rapid fall in viscosity and a disappearance of the filaments. It is evident that neutralization of phage T4 by the lipocarbohydrate involves liberation of nucleic acid from the phage particle.

Extraction of the lipocarbohydrate with 70% ethanol removes some lipid material and renders the hapten inactive in phage neutralization. The activity can be restored by again adding the extracted lipid or by adding myristic, palmitic, or stearic acids. Lower fatty acids or various triglycerides were inactive. Addition of fatty acids to various other polysaccharides did not result in phage-neutralizing activity, suggesting that the activity depended on certain fatty acids adsorbed to a specific polysaccharide.

A given amount of lipocarbohydrate will destroy only a limited number of phage particles, suggesting that the lipocarbohydrate is bound to the phage debris. No evidence was found that the phage liberated dialysable saccharides from the carbohydrate.

Summary of Phage Work

Infection of the host cell by the phages of the T2 serological group involves attachment of the phage tail to the bacterial surface. Primary attachment is electrostatic, facilitated by certain ionic environments, and reversible. Under appropriate conditions this primary attachment is followed by an irreversible step which involves liberation of nucleic acid from the phage particle. Depending on conditions, this nucleic acid may be liberated into the medium with destruction of infectivity, or may enter the host cell with establishment of the vegetative or reproductive state. The release of phage nucleic acid may be brought about by lipopolysaccharide isolated from the host-cell membrane, and even by cation exchange resins indicating that this step is not dependent on host-cell enzymes. Conversely, the phage particle has a marked effect on the host cell which is independent of infection, as demonstrated by the phenomenon of lysis from without. This is undoubtedly an enzymatic reaction but whether it involves an enzyme in the host cell, in the phage particle, or in both is unknown. In all probability the enzyme system involved in lysis from without also functions in the penetration of phage nucleic acid into the host cell. The bacterial receptor site for phage attachment is a lipopolysaccharide. The relationship between this lipopolysaccharide and the enzyme system involved in lysis from without is completely obscure at present.

III. INFLUENZA VIRUSES

These viruses are spherical and about 100 mμ in diameter. They contain carbohydrate, lipid, protein, ribose nucleic acid and some desoxyribose nucleic acid. The entodermal cells of the chick chorioallantoic membrane are the usual experimental host cells although ferret and mouse lungs are used for certain experiments. Virus adsorption to these host cells is followed by an eclipse period during which virus cannot be demonstrated in host cells known to be infected, suggesting that a transition from mature virus to vegetative virus occurs as in the case of phage T2. For an excellent review on the growth of the influenza viruses see Henle (26).

The discovery that influenza virus agglutinates red cells (30) furnished a quick and accurate assay method which has made this the best known animal virus. Although the red cell does not support virus multiplication, it makes a good model for the adsorption step of the infection cycle. The adsorption of influenza virus to red cells differs from adsorption to host cells in one remarkable way: it is followed by a spontaneous elution of the virus from the red cell. This elution results from the destruction of the red-cell receptor substance by the eluting enzyme of the virus, and is accompanied by a permanent alteration of the red-cell surface with loss of ability to adsorb the virus (31). The elution process also causes changes in the electrophoretic mobility and serological properties of the red cells.

The eluting enzyme of influenza virus can be destroyed by appropriate heat-treatment without alteration of the hemagglutinating activity. Such heated preparations are called "indicator virus" because they are sensitive indicators of the presence of soluble inhibitors of hemagglutination which are destroyed by the eluting enzyme of unheated virus.

Soluble inhibitors of hemagglutination are widely distributed in such fluids as serum, saliva, tears, ovarian cyst fluid, and urine. These inhibitors are mucoproteins and are physiologically similar to the receptor substances on the surfaces of erythrocytes and host cells to which the virus adsorbs. The inhibitors are destroyed by the viral eluting enzyme and by the receptor-destroying enzyme of the cholera vibrio.

Receptor-destroying enzyme (RDE) is produced by a variety of bacterial species, the usual source being the cholera vibrio. It appears to be a hydrolytic enzyme and is dependent on calcium ion for its activity. RDE acts upon red cells to render them inagglutinable by influenza virus and alters the red-cell surface as indicated by a change in serological specificity and a less negative electric charge. RDE removes the receptor substance from the surface of host cells and renders them temporarily more resistant to infection with influenza virus. RDE rapidly destroys the ability of mucoproteins to inhibit hemagglutination by indicator virus. As far as comparative experiments have gone, the action of RDE is very similar to that of the viral eluting enzyme (6). The chemical nature of the receptor substance and the mode of action of RDE are challenging problems.

Adsorption of Influenza Virus

The adsorption of influenza virus to a suitable suspension of red cells is a very rapid and efficient process. Calculations by Lanni and Lanni (40), using adsorption data of Hirst (31) and the mathematical analysis that had been applied to phage adsorption, indicated that the rate-limiting factor was the diffusion of the virus. Experimental determination of the adsorption-rate constant by Sagik, Puck, and Levine (52) agreed within a factor of two with the rate calculated on theoretical grounds by Lanni and Lanni (40). However, the discussion of the relative adsorption-rate constants for phage T2 and for influenza virus by Sagik, Puck, and Levine is inapplicable, because the adsorption-rate constant is proportional to the radius of the adsorbing cell, not to its area.

The low temperature coefficient and the marked dependence on salt concentration are in agreement with the high efficiency of adsorption in suggesting that primary attachment of influenza virus to the red-cell surface is by ionic forces. Adsorption to a cation exchange resin is also salt dependent and under appropriate conditions the virus can be eluted in undamaged condition (47). Primary attachment of virus to red cells is readily reversible at 4°C by change of salt concentration (19) or by the addition of cation exchange resin (50). The desorption at 4°C apparently leaves the red-cell surface undamaged and therefore is quite different from the spontaneous elution occurring at higher temperatures which leaves a permanently altered red-cell surface.

The primary attachment of influenza virus to the red-cell surface is very similar to the first step in the adsorption of phage T2 to its host cell. However, the second step in adsorption differs in several ways from the second step in phage adsorption. There is no evidence in the case of phage T2 of an eluting enzyme such as that which is so prominent a feature of influenza virus. Contact of influenza virus with the red-cell membrane, with soluble inhibitor, or with cation exchange resins causes no alteration in the virus properties, in contrast to the case of phage T2 in which similar contacts result in prompt liberation of the phage nucleic acid.

The primary stage in the adsorption of influenza virus to the allantoic membrane appears to be as rapid and efficient as to the red-cell surface. Following this stage most of the adsorbed virus particles progress to a second stage at which they can no longer be detected by infectivity or by serological methods. A small portion of the adsorbed virus remains on the cell surface, from which it may be liberated by the action of RDE. About 30% of the virus inoculum remains apparently unadsorbed, probably because of the action of the eluting enzyme. Virus which has been heated to destroy the eluting enzyme appears to be completely adsorbed (35).

Further evidence that the primary step in adsorption of virus to red cells is essentially the same as to allantoic cells is derived from experiments in which the allantoic cells have been poisoned with azide (33) or with formalin (56). Apparently the second stage is prevented in these poisoned cells because the adsorbed virus elutes again as it does from red cells.

Penetration by Influenza Virus

Following its attachment to the allantoic membrane the major portion of the adsorbed virus disappears and cannot be recovered by treatment of the membrane with RDE or by destruction of the cells. Attempts to recover virus activity as measured by infectivity, hemagglutinin, complement fixing antigen, interfering activity, or immunizing activity have consistently resulted in failure (36). Virus activity cannot be detected for the first two hours of the latent period following infection.

In most respects this resembles the situation during the eclipse period of phage T2 infection but there is one important difference. The phage T2 protein can be demonstrated to remain at the host-cell surface by both isotopic and serological techniques. In contrast, the influenza virus antigen disappears from the surface of the infected host cell and is unable to adsorb antibody when infected allantoic membranes are bathed with diluted antiserum (15, 34). Presumably the entire virus particle penetrates within the host cell, instead of just the nucleic acid as in the case of phage T2.

The mechanism of penetration is still obscure but some suggestive evidence is available. Influenza virus which had been heated to destroy the eluting enzyme but not enough to inhibit hemagglutination adsorbed and penetrated into the cells of the allantois as judged by the disappearance of its ability to absorb antibodies from serum (15, 36). This indicates that the penetration of influenza virus into the host cell is not dependent on the integrity of the eluting enzyme. The fact that active influenza virus does not penetrate into host cells which have been poisoned by formalin or azide strongly suggests that virus penetration is dependent on the activity of host-cell enzymes (33, 56). Penetration of the virus thus seems to be an active process on the part of the host cell, a process termed 'viropexis' by Fazekas (15).

Soluble Receptor Substance

This topic has been extensively discussed in an admirable review by Burnet (9) so that much of the background literature need not be referred to here.

The best preparations of soluble inhibitor so far reported were isolated from human urine by Tamm and Horsfall (57). This material was homogeneous electrophoretically and in the ultracentrifuge and had a molecular weight of about seven million. On hydrolysis the material yielded 33% reducing sugar and 9% glucosamine. Analyses on purified urinary mucoprotein by Gottschalk (21) and Odin (48) gave 5% galactose, 3% mannose, 8% hexosamine, and 1% fucose. In addition Odin found 9% "sialic acid" to be present. This is a crstalline monobasic reducing acid of composition approximating $C_{14}H_{24}NO_{11}$, which gives a purple color with Ehrlich's reagent. Because of the general occurrence of this substance among inhibitory mucoproteins, Odin suggested that it might bear some relation to the receptor substance of erythrocytes. Following this suggestion Gottschalk (22) announced that the prosthetic group of the soluble inhibitors contained 2-carboxy-pyrrole which has some of the properties of sialic acid and may be part of this acid. He suggested that in the mucoproteins the —COOH of the pyrrole may be in amide linkage with hexosamine and the imino group may be in glycosidic linkage with a sugar. Treatment of soluble inhibitor with either virus or RDE results in liberation of a dialysable component containing carbohydrate and the carboxy-pyrrole. The residual mucoprotein is less negatively charged, is not detectably altered in sedimentation rate (57), and has an increased viscosity (12). It no longer is able to inhibit hemagglutination by indicator virus but retains its serological activity. These results are consistent with the assumption that the eluting enzyme and RDE are amidases hydrolysing the amide link between the carboxy-pyrrole and a hexosamine to liberate a low molecular fragment (23).

The effects of periodate are also consistent with this picture of the receptor substance. Periodate is a potent oxidizing agent which oxidizes many substances including compounds such as glycols and sugars which have alcohol groups on adjacent carbons. Treatment of red cells with suitable concentrations of periodate will destroy their ability to absorb the influenza viruses (32). Treatment with lower concentrations will not interfere with the adsorption of virus, but the virus is now unable to elute, and cannot be removed by treatment with RDE. This adsorbed virus is still active as far as its effect on normal red cells is concerned (16). Periodate has a similar modifying effect *in vivo* on the virus receptors of mouse lung and chick allantois. Nevertheless, influenza virus is able to infect such modified host cells, suggesting again that infection may occur in the absence of detectable activity on the part of the eluting enzyme, in this case because the substrate has been chemically modified so that it cannot be attacked by the enzymes (16). Periodate-treated mucoproteins are able to inhibit active influenza viruses in the same way that untreated mucoids inhibit indicator virus; however, the inhibition by periodate-treated mucoids is not reversed by treatment with RDE as in the case of mucoid inhibition of indicator virus (8). These results suggest that periodate-treated receptor substance can still combine with the enzymes but it has been so altered chemically that it is no longer a substrate; it behaves like the class of enzyme inhibitors which are structural analogues of the usual substrates. This is in part the basis for Gottschalk's suggestion that the carboxy-pyrrole is linked to a hexosamine, the hexosamine being the periodate-sensitive component of the receptor substance. Periodate damage to the hexosamine might be close enough to the hydrolyzable bond to interfere with enzyme action. This interpretation is reasonable but by no means conclusive.

Role of Intracellular Receptor Substance

Although the eluting enzyme seems to play no role in the penetration of the virus into the host cell, it is still possible, as suggested by Burnet (9) and others, that it may be involved in the intracellular development of the virus. Experiments by Isaacs and Edney (37) on intracellular interference by heated influenza virus with the multiplication of various strains of active virus seemed to show that the ability of a strain of active virus "to overcome competitively" the interference was correlated with its position in the receptor gradient. This was interpreted as evidence that intracellular receptor substance played some role in virus development, the heated interfering virus competing with active virus for attachment to the receptors on nucleo-protein synthesizing sites in the host cell. However, careful quantitative experiments by Fazekas and Edney (17) demonstrated quite conclusively that infection of an allantoic cell by a single heated virus particle was sufficient to prevent completely the multiplication of active virus in that cell regardless of the dose of active virus used. The explanation for the discrepancy between these two papers is the time interval between addition of heated, interfering virus and active virus, 1 hr in the experiments of Isaacs and Edney, 24 hr in those of Fazekas and Edney. Interference does not become established in all cells for some time following adsorption of virus (18).

A recent preliminary report by Schlesinger (54) reopened the question of a possible role of intracellular receptor substance and of the eluting enzyme in virus multiplication. Eggs were inoculated by the allantoic route with enough influenza virus to infect all entodermal cells. At intervals during virus growth membranes were removed, pooled, and aliquots were assayed separately for hemagglutinating activity (virus) and for hemagglutinin inhibiting activity (intracellular receptor substance). During the period when intracellular hemagglutinin was increasing rapidly, there was a large decrease in intracellular receptor substance as had been noted previously by Liu and Henle (42). This indicates that the eluting enzyme is active in destroying receptor substance during the period of active virus multiplication, and that the substrate must be in contact with the enzyme in the intracellular environment. The surprising event was that during the succeeding period, while the intracellular level of hemagglutinin remained constant, the concentration of intracellular receptor substance increased, only to fall a second time during the next rise in virus level. Because this cyclic fluctuation in concentration of intracellular receptor substance appeared to be correlated with the cycles of virus growth, Schlesinger (55) suggested that the destruction of intracellular receptor substance by the virus enzyme may play an essential role in virus multiplication, perhaps as a source of raw material. More direct evidence in support of this interesting hypothesis will undoubtedly be sought. Meanwhile, there seems to be no clear-cut evidence for concluding that intracellular receptor substance plays an essential role in virus multiplication, or that the eluting enzyme has any function other than that of destroying extracellular inhibitor to facilitate virus adsorption to the host cell.

Summary of Influenza Work

Primary attachment of influenza virus to the surface of red cells and host cells involves electrostatic forces and is readily reversible. Under appropriate conditions attachment of influenza virus to red cells is followed by spontaneous elution, the result of damage to the receptor substance by a virus enzyme. Attachment of influenza virus to host cells is followed by penetration of the entire virus particle into the host cell. This penetration is independent of the activity of the eluting enzyme of the virus and appears to involve an active process on the part of the host cell. Most animal fluids contain soluble mucoproteins which are chemically and physiologically very similar to the receptor substances on red cells and host cells. These soluble receptor substances competitively interfere with attachment of virus to red cells and host cells. Under conditions in which the virus-eluting enzyme is nonfunctional the soluble receptor substances completely prevent attachment of virus to red cell and host cell by occupying the attachment sites on the virus particles.

It seems evident that in nature the influenza virus would be unable to perpetuate itself if it lacked the eluting enzyme, because the soluble receptor substance in respiratory mucus would effectively prevent contact of the virus particles with their usual host cells (9). This would seem to be sufficient explanation for the retention of the eluting enzyme system during the evolutionary development of the influenza viruses. In any event, attempts to demonstrate a role for this enzyme in virus penetration, or in intracellular virus multiplication, have so far resulted in failure, so its only known role is the destruction of extracellular receptor substance.

Conclusions

The role of host-cell polysaccharides in the reproduction of bacteriophage T2 and influenza virus seems to be solely that of furnishing a chemically specific site to which the virus particles become attached as the first step of the infection cycle. In the case of phage T2, attachment of the virus particle to the receptor polysaccharide is immediately followed by release of the phage nucleic acid from the protein membrane of the particle. Depending on environmental circumstances the phage nucleic acid may then either enter into the host cell or be released into the suspending medium. Although the phage particle can disrupt bacterial cells by the process known as "lysis from without," it is not known whether the enzymes involved are part of the host cell or part of the phage particle. There is no evidence that the host polysaccharides are substrates for these lytic enzymes.

In the case of influenza virus, attachment to a synthetically competent

host cell is followed by penetration of the entire virus particle into the cell
interior. If the virus attaches to an incompetent host cell such as an erythro-
cyte or a poisoned cell, the viral eluting enzyme liberates the virus particle
in undamaged condition. If the virus becomes attached to soluble receptor
substance, the viral enzyme destroys the inhibitory activity of the receptor
substance and liberates the virus particle to try again to find a suitable
host cell. There is no evidence that the eluting enzyme plays a role in penetration or intracellular multiplication of the virus.

The chemical structure of the receptor polysaccharides is responsible for
host-cell specificity in virus infections, insofar as susceptibility is dependent
upon adsorption of virus to cell. Whether infection results in the production of virus progeny depends on factors other than the presence of a
specific host-cell polysaccharide.

REFERENCES

1. Adams, M. H. (1954). Dynamics of Virus Infection. Symposium of the Henry
   Ford Hospital, Detroit.
2. Anderson, T. F. (1945). *J. Cellular Comp. Physiol.* 25, 1.
3. Anderson, T. F. (1945). *J. Cellular Comp. Physiol.* 25, 17.
4. Anderson, T. F. (1951). *Trans. N. Y. Acad. Sci.* 13, 130.
5. Boivin, A. (1946). *Schweiz. Z. Pathol. u. Bacteriol.* 9, 506.
6. Briody, B. A. (1948). *J. Immunol.* 59, 115.
7. Burnet, F. M. (1930). *J. Pathol. Bacteriol.* 33, 647.
8. Burnet, F. M. (1949). *Australian J. Exptl. Biol. Med. Sci.* 27, 361.
9. Burnet, F. M. (1951). *Physiol. Revs.* 31, 131.
10. Burnet, F. M., Keogh, E. V., and Lush, D. (1937). *Australian J. Exptl. Biol. Med.
    Sci.* 15, 227.
11. Cohen, S. S. (1949). *Bacteriol. Revs.* 13, 1.
12. Curtain, C. C. (1953). *Australian J. Exptl. Biol. Med. Sci.* 31, 255.
13. Delbruck, M. (1940). *J. Gen. Physiol.* 23, 643.
14. Doermann, A. H. (1953). *Cold Spring Harbor Symposia Quant. Biol.* 18, 3.
15. Fazekas de St. Groth, S. (1948). *Nature* 162, 294.
16. Fazekas de St. Groth, S. (1949). *Australian J. Exptl. Biol. Med. Sci.* 27, 65.
17. Fazekas de St. Groth, S. and Edney, M. (1952). *J. Immunol.* 69, 160.
18. Fazekas de St. Groth, S., Isaacs, A., and Edney, M. (1952). *Nature* 170, 573.
19. Flick, J. A., Sanford, B., and Mudd, S. (1949). *J. Immunol.* 61, 65.
20. Goebel, W. F. (1950). *J. Exptl. Med.* 92, 527.
21. Gottschalk, A. (1952). *Nature* 170, 662.
22. Gottschalk, A. (1953). *Nature* 172, 808.
23. Gottschalk, A. (1954). Dynamics of Virus Infection, Symposium of the Henry
    Ford Hospital, Detroit.
24. Graham, A. F. (1953). *Ann. inst. Pasteur* 84, 90.
25. Heagy, F. C. (1950). *J. Bacteriol.* 59, 367.
26. Henle, W. (1953). *Advances in Virus Research* 1, 141.
27. Herriott, R. M. (1951). *J. Bacteriol.* 61, 752.
28. Hershey, A. D. and Chase, M. (1952). *J. Gen. Physiol.* 36, 39.

29. Hershey, A. D., Kalmanson, G., and Bronfenbrenner, J. (1944). *J. Immunol.* 48, 221.
30. Hirst, G. K. (1941). *Science* 94, 22.
31. Hirst, G. K. (1942). *J. Exptl. Med.* 76, 195.
32. Hirst, G. K. (1948). *J. Exptl. Med.* 87, 301.
33. Hoyle, L. (1948). *Brit. J. Exptl. Pathol.* 29, 390.
34. Hoyle, L. (1950). *J. Hyg.* 48, 277.
35. Isaacs, A. and Edney, M. (1950*a*). *Australian J. Exptl. Biol. Med. Sci.* 28, 231.
36. Isaacs, A. and Edney, M. (1950*b*). *Australian J. Exptl. Biol. Med. Sci.* 28, 635.
37. Isaacs, A. and Edney, M. (1951). *Australian J. Exptl. Biol. Med. Sci.* 29, 169, 179.
38. Jesaitis, M. and Goebel, W. F. (1952). *J. Exptl. Med.* 96, 425.
39. Jesaitis, M. and Goebel, W. F. (1953). *Cold Spring Harbor Symposia Quant. Biol.* 18, 205.
40. Lanni, F. and Lanni, Y. T. (1952). *J. Bacteriol.* 64, 865.
41. Lark, K. G. and Adams, M. H. (1953). *Cold Spring Harbor Symposia Quant. Biol.* 18, 171.
42. Liu, O. C. and Henle, W. (1951). *J. Exptl. Med.* 94, 269.
43. Luria, S. E. (1945). *Genetics* 30, 84.
44. Miller, E. M. and Goebel, W. F. (1949). *J. Exptl. Med.* 90, 255.
45. Monod, J. and Wollman, E. (1947). *Ann. inst. Pasteur* 73, 937.
46. Morgan, W. T. J. (1949). The Nature of the Bacterial Surface. Blackwell Scientific Publications, Oxford.
47. Muller, R. H. and Rose, H. M. (1952). *Proc. Soc. Exptl. Biol. Med.* 80, 27.
48. Odin, L. (1952). *Nature* 170, 663.
49. Puck, T. T. (1953). *Cold Spring Harbor Symposia Quant. Biol.* 18, 149.
50. Puck, T. T. and Sagik, B. (1953). *J. Exptl. Med.* 97, 807.
51. Puck, T. T., Garen, A., and Cline, J. (1951). *J. Exptl. Med.* 93, 65.
52. Sagik, B., Puck, T., and Levine, S. (1954). *J. Exptl. Med.* 99, 251.
53. Schlesinger, M. (1932). *Z. Hyg. Infektionskrankh.* 114, 130.
54. Schlesinger, R. W. (1953*a*). *Proc. 6th Intern. Congr. Microbiol.* (Roma), Symp. on Interaction of Viruses and Cells, p. 36.
55. Schlesinger, R. W. (1953*b*). *Cold Spring Harbor Symposia Quant. Biol.* 18, 55.
56. Stone, J. D. (1948). *Australian J. Exptl. Biol. Med. Sci.* 26, 49, 287.
57. Tamm, I. and Horsfall, F. L. (1952). *J. Exptl. Med.* 95, 71.
58. Tolmach, L. J. and Puck, T. T. (1952). *J. Am. Chem. Soc.* 74, 5551.
59. Visconti, N. (1953). *J. Bacteriol.* 66, 247.
60. Watson, J. D. (1950). *J. Bacteriol.* 60, 697.
61. Weidel, W. (1951). *Z. Naturforsch.* 6b, 251.
62. Weidel, W. (1953). *Cold Spring Harbor Symposia. Quant. Biol.* 18, 155.
63. Weidel, W. (1953). *Ann. inst. Pasteur* 84, 60.

SOME METABOLIC AND CYTOCHEMICAL ASPECTS OF BACTERIOPHAGE INFECTION

By S. E. Luria, *University of Illinois, Urbana, Illinois*

I. INTRODUCTION

In considering fundamental aspects of viral infections we are dealing with the functional organization, normal or abnormal, of the cell. Two contradictory aspects of viral infection at the cellular level—integration and destructiveness—must be considered and distinguished from epiphenomena, representing more or less specific reactions to the primary cellular alterations. The possibility of analyzing the viral infection of isolated, noninteracting cells such as bacteria has been responsible for the outstanding success of bacteriophage research.

Phage research is dominated today by three main concepts:

1. We accept a dual structure and function of infectious phage, as a reproductive and controlling core consisting mainly of desoxyribonucleic acid (=DNA) and a protein apparatus functional in external infection but reproductively dispensable.

2. We accept a functional and probably physical integration of phage, in its *prophage* (=latent) form, with the hereditary apparatus of the bacterial cell.

3. We visualize the production of infectious (i.e., transmissible) phage as an accessory, if indispensable, aspect of phage-bacterium relation.

Recent publications (24, 21) contain the justification for the above statements, which will serve as a background for our rapid survey of metabolic aspects of phage-bacterium relations. This survey will be directed to listing areas of actual or potential interest rather than to detailing our present knowledge.

We shall deal with three aspects of phage-bacterium relationship. First, we shall consider effects of the metabolic state of the host on the outcome of exogenous phage attacks. Second, we shall mention effects of established prophages on metabolic functions of lysogenic bacteria. Third, we shall discuss certain aspects of the vegetative reproduction of phage and of its maturation into the infectious form.

132

II. HOST METABOLISM AND RESPONSE TO PHAGE INFECTION

Nutritional and metabolic factors influence the outcome of phage-bacterium interaction. A brief listing will show the wide potentialities of this approach.

1. Resistant bacterial mutants fail either to adsorb phage or to carry out the irreversible phases of attachment. Nutritional deficiencies coupled with acquisition of resistance have never been assessed adequately in relation to virus susceptibility. Occasionally, a "resistant" mutant will adsorb phage and be killed if its cells have reached nutritional starvation (20).

2. Abortive phage infection has been observed in many instances: with bacteria suddenly transferred to anaerobiosis or otherwise blocked in utilization of available energy sources (4, 8); with bacteria receiving phage restricted in its growth potential by previous growth in different hosts (18); with bacteria carrying certain unrelated prophages (see below). These abortive infections result in normal adsorption (and sometimes death of the host) with failure of virus development in the great majority of the cells. The significant lead is that the minority proportion of bacterial cells in which phage succeeds in growing can be increased (often from 1 in 10^4 to 1 in 10 or more) by pre-exposure of the host bacteria to a variety of nutritional or metabolic conditions, specific for each system (starvation; poisoning by fermentation products; amino-acid analogues; energy-uncoupling agents; radiation). Thus, internal inhibitions to phage development can be overcome by various treatments.

3. The outcome of infection with a temperate phage, either into lysogenicity or into phage multiplication and lysis, is also subject to environmental and biochemical control (3, 21). Temperature, metabolic poisons, and special nutrients, applied before or after infection, can shift the relative frequencies of the two alternative results.

III. THE PHYSIOLOGICAL ROLE OF PROPHAGE

This most intriguing aspect of phage-bacterium interaction includes effects at various levels:

1. Immunity of a lysogenic bacterium to lysis by phage related to its own prophage (except for its supervirulent mutants) may result directly from the presence of the prophage material at critical locations in the lysogenic cells, presumably in the chromosomal apparatus.

2. Interference by a prophage with multiplication of unrelated phages, resulting in abortive infection (2), may be the expression of a metabolic role of prophage, since it is influenced by a variety of external metabolic agencies (17). A prophage may also control the ability of the bacterial

cell to induce temporary, phenotypic modifications in certain unrelated phages (1).

3. The control of toxin production by prophage in *Corynebacterium diphtheriae* (7) is certainly a metabolic effect. All toxigenic strains are lysogenic, and nontoxigenic strains can be made toxigenic by lysogenization.

In studying effects of this type, it will be well to visualize them as expressions of the genome of the lysogenic cell considered as an integrated whole rather than as the sum of two independently working moieties—the prophage and the host genome.

IV. THE SYNTHESIS OF INFECTIOUS VIRUS

Infectious phage may develop either soon after infection (*lytic infection*) or, in lysogenic bacteria, after spontaneous or induced "activation" of the prophage. Vegetative reproduction of phage in noninfectious form is followed by maturation into infectious form.

1. As for host-specific constituents, we encounter a variety of situations:

a. In some systems (T group of coli-phages) the synthesis of many host-specific constituents is arrested. Pre-existing enzymes continue to operate and provide the materials and energy needed for phage synthesis (4).

b. In other systems, syntheses of host constituents continue until the time of lysis alongside with phage specific synthesis (21). Yet, at least one instance of keen competition between the two processes has been observed, phage synthesis being preferentially spared when the carbon source supply becomes limiting for residual host syntheses (11).

2. Concerning phage-specific syntheses, work on coli-phages of the T2 group permits us to distinguish several levels:

a. At the level of low-molecular-weight constituents, there is, on the one hand, a change in carbohydrate metabolism with desoxyribose synthesis favored over ribose synthesis. This change is secondary to the arrest in RNA synthesis (5). On the other hand, phage infection forces the synthesis of a unique, phage-specific pyrimidine (hydroxymethyl cytosine) in bacteria that, when uninfected, neither produce it nor utilize it. Also, synthesis of thymine can be forced by phage in a "thymineless" organism (5).

b. Phage DNA (characterized for T-even phages by having hydroxymethyl cytosine instead of cytosine) is synthesized at an approximately constant rate (10), being assembled from a pool fed by new syntheses and by a specific breakdown of host DNA. Synthesis of DNA may be forced by phage infection upon cells that had been made unable to form DNA by certain treatments [mustard gas, (9); radiations, (13)]. There is evidence (14) for the activation by phage infection of a powerful DNA-ase, probably by removal of a normally present inhibitor; the degradation of host DNA, to be made available into the pool, may be a result of activation of DNA-ase. Some observations suggest that there may be little or no contribution of materials from host proteins to phage proteins, an indication that the degradation of host DNA is not just a result of an overall degradation of host constituents. Cytological observations have demonstrated the selective, specific disintegration of organized DNA structures in bacteria infected with the T phages.

Hence, phage infection seems to emerge as a nuclear pathology, more specifically, as strictly a DNA pathology. It may be that those host syntheses that are suppressed by the T phages require a more or less direct intervention of the cell DNA.

Although no analytical distinction can yet be made between host DNA and viral DNA in phage systems other than the T-even phages, the concept of a DNA pathology may well be one of general validity. A temporary delay in DNA synthesis is observed in infection with temperate phages (21). Cytologically, several temperate phages produce characteristic, profound, though reversible nuclear alterations. The interference by a prophage with the development of an unrelated phage may reflect a specific resistance of the prophage-containing DNA system to certain DNA intruders.

c. As for phage proteins, serological evidence indicates that their appearance and increase precede by a few minutes and parallel the appearance and increase of infectious phage (16). Over-all increase in protein before the rise in phage antigens, in instances where host enzymes fail to be formed (4), may hold the key to the discovery of unsuspected early events in phage development.

Little is known about the mechanism of phage protein synthesis. Excess phage antigens (as well as excess DNA) are liberated along with infectious phage. There is no evidence for any phage-specific machinery in protein synthesis as distinct from the specificity-imparting control (DNA?). A remarkable expression of phage control over the synthesis of its own proteins is the occurrence of normal phage development in bacteria that have received enough ultraviolet light to suppress synthesis of adaptive enzymes (12).

3. In the formation of infectious phage, work on T-even phages provides circumstantial evidence for a distinct process of assembly of phage constituents into the final product—the infectious particle. This evidence includes, first, the presence of two major protein components, the sero-

logically distinct "head" and "tail" proteins (15), as separate entities before and alongside mature phage; second, the finding that all major phage components (DNA, head and tail proteins) are produced in normal amounts, but separate from each other, under the influence of proflavine (6); and third, the existence of phenotypic mixing. Phenotypic mixing is the formation, in mixed-infected bacteria, of phage particles whose serological and host range properties do not match their hereditary properties (22). An analysis of phenotypic mixing (23) suggests a random association of phage elements (presumably DNA cores) of any given genotype with tail protein of any one type formed in a given bacterium.

An appealing picture is one according to which phage DNA reproduces in the form of extended fibers and controls, directly or indirectly, the synthesis of specific phage proteins. There follows a coiling of the long DNA fibers (about 2×10^6 Å in phage T2) into the condensed phage core (about 500 Å diameter), coupled with a crystallization of the phage proteins into the surrounding shell and appended tail. The presence in the shell of one particle of proteins with specificity corresponding to other phage cores indicates a dualism between protein synthesis and protein assembly. The coupling of phage with random fragments of host DNA, evidenced by transduction phenomena in Salmonella, may take place either during the reproductive process or upon assembly of the phage.

V. CONCLUSION

Phage infection of a bacterial cell is envisioned as a change in function, resulting from addition or substitution of new specificity-controlling patterns. Metabolically speaking, the phage-infected cell may be considered as a stable or self-destructive mutant of the uninfected cell. Time will tell whether this picture fits other virus infections as well. We now recognize several types of infectious heredity, resulting in functionally integrated systems. The question may well be asked whether virus infection may not simply recapitulate the early process of the origin of cells.

REFERENCES

1. Anderson, E. S. and Felix, A. (1953). *J. Gen. Microbiol.* 8, 408.
2. Bertani, G. (1953). *Cold Spring Harbor Symposia Quant. Biol.* 18, 65.
3. Bertani, G. and Nice, S. J. (1954). *J. Bacteriol.* 67, 202.
4. Cohen, S. S. (1949). *Bacteriol. Revs.* 13, 1.
5. Cohen, S. S. (1953). *Cold Spring Harbor Symposia Quant. Biol.* 18, 221.
6. De Mars, R. I., Luria, S. E., Fisher, H., and Levinthal, C. (1953). *Ann. inst. Pasteur* 84, 113.
7. Freeman, V. J. and Morse, I. U. (1952). *J. Bacteriol.* 63, 407.
8. Heagy, F. C. (1950). *J. Bacteriol.* 59, 367.
9. Herriott, R. M. (1951). *J. Gen. Physiol.* 34, 761.

10. Hershey, A. D., Dixon, J., and Chase, M. (1953). *J. Gen. Physiol.* 36, 777.
11. Jacob, F. (1953). *Ann. inst. Pasteur* 84, 254.
12. Jacob, F., Torriani, A.-M., and Monod, J. (1951). *Compt. rend.* 233, 1230.
13. Kelner, A. (1953). *J. Bacteriol.* 65, 252.
14. Kozloff, L. M. (1953). *Cold Spring Harbor Symposia Quant. Biol.* 18, 207.
15. Lanni, F. and Lanni, Y. T. (1953). *Cold Spring Harbor Symposia Quant. Biol.* 18, 159.
16. Lanni, Y. T. (1954). *J. Bacteriol.* 67, 640.
17. Lederberg, S. (1953). Unpublished results.
18. Luria, S. E. (1953). *Cold Spring Harbor Symposia Quant. Biol.* 18, 237.
19. Luria, S. E. and Human, M. L. (1950). *J. Bacteriol.* 59, 551.
20. Luria, S. E. and Human, M. L. (1952). *J. Bacteriol.* 64, 557.
21. Lwoff, A. (1953). *Bacteriol. Revs.* 17, 269.
22. Novick, A. and Szilard, L. (1951). *Science* 113, 34.
23. Streisinger, G. (1953). Ph. D. Thesis, University of Illinois.
24. (1953). Viruses. *Cold Spring Harbor Symposia Quant. Biol.* 18.
25. Zinder, N. D. (1953). *Cold Spring Harbor Symposia Quant. Biol.* 18, 261.

METABOLISM OF INFECTED CELLS

By E. Racker,* *Department of Biochemistry, Yale University School of Medicine*

I. GENERAL CONSIDERATIONS

We consider viruses to be living organisms. They are living in the sense that they contain a genetic apparatus which permits them to struggle for survival—if you wish to call that living. Since they exist within cells, politely called the hosts, viruses are parasites, whether they originated from within or from without. They contain no enzyme system which can provide utilizable energy. They live therefore at the expense of the host who may be destroyed in the process. This life and death struggle is called "the virus-host relationship" in the gentle language of the virologist. The virus usually wins either by killing the host or by making his life miserable in the cold war of lysogenicity.

The infected cell is metabolically an altered cell. Changes of nucleic-acid metabolism in infected bacteria (5), of carbohydrate metabolism in infected animal tissues (17), and of protein metabolism of infected plant tissues (2) have been reported. The infected cell synthesizes new virus protein and nucleic acid—a process in which it may deprive itself of nutrients and energy which are required for the synthesis of its own constituents (10). The infected cell may exhibit new synthetic ability in pyrimidine metabolism (6) and numerous quantitative alterations in various enzyme activities have been recorded. Since these have been reviewed elsewhere (1), they will not be discussed here. Instead, an attempt will be made to point to some of the difficulties which have been encountered in studies of the metabolism of infected cells and to evaluate what may be learned from such an approach.

1. Difficulties of Experimental Approach and Choice of System

First, it is necessary to select an infected cell population that is suitable for metabolic studies. There can be little doubt that bacteria infected with the incomparable bacteriophages offer many advantages: considerable uniformity of host cells and viruses, reasonably accurate assay methods, ease

* Present address: The Public Health Research Institute of the City of New York, New York 21, N. Y.

138

of controlling multiplicity of infection, environmental conditions, etc. On the other hand, the metabolic complexity of the bacterial host cell which can synthesize all its cellular constituents from glucose or lactate as the only carbon source is a distinct disadvantage and presents numerous experimental difficulties of analysis. Thus the investigator is forced to search for a thin metabolic trail left by the virus in the forest of metabolism.

If infected plant or animal tissues are chosen for metabolic studies, the disadvantages appear obvious: difficulties of evaluating quantitative aspects of the infectious process; lack of cellular uniformity of the host tissue, which may contain susceptible as well as resistant cells; the complication of secondary inflammatory changes; etc. In an organ such as the brain, damage to a small but vital center may produce an effect which is out of proportion to the extent of the infectious process. However, one great advantage of choosing brain tissue for such studies is the fact that, metabolically speaking, brain is the land of sugar and honey. Brain metabolism is characterized by a predominance of carbohydrate catabolism, as shown by the respiratory quotient of unity. Although for virus multiplication protein and nucleic acid synthesis are undoubtedly essential, the energy supply must come from the breakdown of carbohydrates, a process that is also essential for the maintenance of brain function. In view of our rather extensive knowledge of carbohydrate metabolism, an alteration can be readily detected and analyzed.

2. Difficulties of Interpretation

Let us suppose we have made an observation of a change in metabolism in an infected cell population. We are now faced with new problems. What part does this metabolic change play in the infectious process, either in the multiplication of the virus or in the destruction of the host cell? What are the chances of ascribing a metabolic variation in a multienzyme system to a well-defined enzyme reaction? Will the localization of the defect help us to explain the mechanism responsible for its appearance?

Rather than attempt to give general answers to these questions, two examples have been selected which will illustrate difficulties of experimental approach as well as of interpretation. The first example deals with the nucleic acid metabolism of infected *E. coli* cells, the second with the carbohydrate metabolism of infected brain tissue.

II. METABOLIC ALTERATIONS IN INFECTED BACTERIA

It was reported seven years ago (5) that, in *E. coli* strain B infected with T2 bacteriophage, the net synthesis of both ribose nucleic acid (RNA) and desoxyribose nucleic acid (DNA) ceases abruptly. After an apparent lag period, synthesis of DNA is resumed as show in Fig 1. No net synthesis of RNA can be detected. This dramatic metabolic alteration can be brought about by a single virus particle which, in fact, need not be infectious, since phage irradiated with ultraviolet light produces a similar effect.

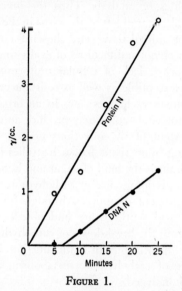

FIGURE 1.

These findings were confirmed in several laboratories. In Fig. 2 an experiment is shown which demonstrates the effect of ultraviolet irradiated bacteriophage on bacterial synthesis of nucleic acids (20). Since these measurements were made spectrophotometrically at 260 mµ, it is clear that infection with heavily irradiated phage (which does not lead to multiplicity reactivation), inhibits the formation not only of the polynucleotides but also of purines and pyrimidines and other compounds which absorb strongly at this wavelength. Recent studies indicate that the block in RNA metabolism may be incomplete. Hershey (9) demonstrated a limited exchange of inorganic P^{32} with an RNA fraction of *E. coli* during infection with T2, however this may not represent net synthesis of RNA. The investigations of Kozloff (1953) also point to a limited turnover of RNA. In these studies it was shown that an RNA which acts as an inhibitor DNA-ase activity disappears from infected *E. coli* cells, resulting in an apparent increase in DNA-ase activity.

These investigations of alterations in nucleic acid metabolism of infected *E. coli* cells lead to numerous contributions to our knowledge of bacterial nucleic acid and carbohydrate metabolism (cf. 6, 8). They also stimulated the study of the synthesis and breakdown of ribose and desoxyribose phosphate (22, 23) and led to the discovery of a new pyrimidine 5-hydroxymethyl cytosine (cf. 6) which is present in the even-numbered T phages.

Although quantitative alterations in the glucose-6-phosphate oxidation

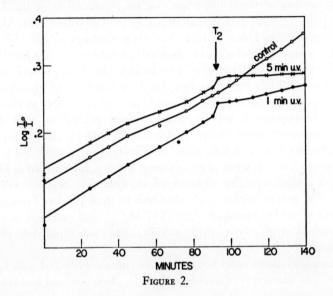

FIGURE 2.

shunt have been observed to follow infections with T2, these minor changes in the synthesis of ribose-5-phosphate do not explain the pronounced inhibition of RNA synthesis. The role of hydroxymethylation of pyrimidine nucleosides in the alteration of nucleic-acid metabolism still remains to be clarified in view of the limited distribution of this base and the more widely encountered changes of nucleic-acid metabolism.

III. METABOLIC ALTERATIONS IN INFECTED BRAIN HOMOGENATES

The second example concerns our own work on the effect of neurotropic viruses on brain metabolism which was carried out at New York University. The investigation had been started over 12 years ago but progressed very slowly. So many difficulties were encountered that the work required continuous encouragement and stimulus, extensive knowledge of intermediary metabolism and organic chemistry, great accuracy of experimentation, a good deal of stubbornness, and infinite patience. I would like to take this opportunity to thank Dr. C. M. MacLeod who supplied the stimulus, Dr. S. Ochoa who contributed his knowledge of intermediary metabolism, Dr. Ratner, Dr. Adams, and Dr. Pappenheimer who advised

in problems of organic chemistry, and to Dr. I. Krimsky who did most of
the experimental work. This leaves for me the stubbornness for which my
wife permitted me to take full credit. She claims for herself the credit of
infinite patience.

Early studies of brain dispersions of mice infected with the Lansing
strain of poliomyelitis indicated an impairment of glycolysis (15). Although
other investigators failed to reproduce these findings in mice (26), they
obtained a similar inhibition of glycolysis in cords of cotton rats infected
with Lansing virus (27). In order to localize the defect, it was necessary
to study the utilization of phosphorylated intermediates of glycolysis. This
was not possible with intact cells which are not permeable to these compounds. Disruption of cell structure by homogenization with distilled
water eliminated permeability problems but unfortunately also eliminated glycolysis. A systematic study of glycolysis in mouse-brain homogenates revealed the presence of an inhibitor which was identified as DPNase
and was counteracted by addition of nicotinamide. Sodium salts were
found to be potent inhibitors of glycolysis in these cell-free homogenates.
Addition of DPN, nicotinamide, ATP, Mg^{++}, and omission of sodium
salts resulted in glycolysis which was 20 times more rapid than observed
with slices (16).

When glycolysis in brain homogenates of animals infected with Lansing
poliomyelitis virus was reinvestigated under these optimal conditions for

TABLE I

INHIBITION OF GLUCOSE UTILIZATION IN INFECTED BRAIN HOMOGENATES

| Virus | Substrate | Number of mouse brains | | Average inhibition of glucose utilization, per cent |
		Normal	Infected	
Lansing	Glucose	36	36	15.0
Lansing	Fructose-1, 6-diphosphate	36	36	3.5
Theiler FA	Glucose	20	24	31.5
Theiler FA	Fructose-1, 6-diphosphate	5	5	4.5

glycolysis, the inhibition was still demonstrable. (Table I). More pronounced and reproducible data than those observed with Lansing virus
were obtained with tissues infected with Theiler FA virus of mouse

encephalomyelitis. The inhibition was apparent with glucose as substrate while addition of fructose-1,6-diphosphate (HDP) eliminated the inhibition. As shown in Table II, the defect was apparent in the rate of glucose disappearance, lactic acid accumulation, and also in the formation of phosphate esters.

TABLE II

INHIBITION OF GLUCOSE UTILIZATION AND PHOSPHATE ESTERIFICATION IN MOUSE-BRAIN HOMOGENATES INFECTED WITH THEILER FA VIRUS

Mouse brain	Change in one hour		
	Glucose, mg	Lactic acid, mg	P-ester mg P
Normal	−1.91	+1.75	+0.196
Infected	−0.1	+0.96	+0.1

The accurate localization of this metabolic defect turned out to be a fascinating exercise in analyzing multienzyme systems. Since lactic-acid production was not impaired with HDP as substrate (Table I), it was at first suspected that one of the enzymes which catalyze the formation of HDP from glucose was inhibited. Therefore hexokinase (3), hexose isomerase, and phosphohexokinase (18), were purified and tested for their capacity to restore glycolysis in infected brain. They proved to be without effect (18). However, a few micrograms of another enzyme fraction obtained from either muscle or yeast were found to restore glycolysis. This "restoring factor" was identified as glyceraldehyde-3-phosphate dehydrogenase. Crystalline preparations of this enzyme effectively restored glycolysis to infected brain homogenates of low glycolytic activity (Table III).

This finding was rather unexpected since glyceraldehyde-3-phosphate dehydrogenase is required for lactic-acid production from either glucose or HDP but utilization of the latter showed little or no impairment in infected tissues. An analysis of this apparent discrepancy revealed that the defect was in the regeneration of ATP which is required for glucose phosphorylation (21). In the presence of ATPase activity, this regeneration process is the limiting factor in brain glycolysis with glucose as the only source of energy. Addition of the phosphocreatine → ATP regenerating system also restored glycolysis to inhibited homogenates.

The next problem was to determine the mode of inactivation of glyceraldehyde-3-phosphate dehydrogenase and the role played by the virus in this process. We were quite pleased to discover that addition of a purified preparation of the FA virus of mouse encephalomyelitis resulted in an

TABLE III

Restoration of Glycolysis by Glyceraldehyde-3-phosphate Dehydrogenase

Mouse-brain homogenate	Lactic acid per hour, mg
Normal brain	2.1
Normal brain + ferrous sulfate	0.3
Normal brain + ferrous sulfate + triose-p-dehydrogenase	2.3
Infected brain	0.6
Infected brain + triose-p-dehydrogenase	2.4

inhibition of glycolysis indistinguishable from that observed in infected tissues. We were less pleased when we found that a boiled virus preparation inhibited also, and we were slightly shocked to find that incinerated virus would do likewise. The inhibiting effect was traced to the iron content of the virus preparation and could be reproduced by traces of ferrous sulfate. Attempts to remove the inhibitory iron from the virus by salt fractionation, electrodialysis, and high-speed centrifugation failed (18). The fact that the iron is firmly bound to the virus but at the same time exerts its inhibitory influence on brain glycolysis suggested the possibility of a metabolic influence of the divalent ion in the infectious process. Other divalent ions have been found in some other viruses, e.g. copper in vaccinia virus, and in some instances have been shown to be needed early in the infectious process, e.g. in T5 infection of E. coli (cf. 13). Lwoff has proposed a stimulating theory in regard to the mode of action and role of divalent ions in the process of molecular reproduction (14).

The mechanism of the inactivation of triose phosphate dehydrogenase was then investigated. The virus—or ferrous salts—were found to activate a heat-labile factor in brain which in turn inactivated the triose phosphate dehydrogenase. A partial purification of the heat-labile brain factor revealed that it required cysteine or ascorbic acid as well as ferrous ions for full activity. Since its effect was on a protein and was reproduced by the addition of purified proteolytic enzymes (12), the possibility was considered that the factor in brain is a proteolytic enzyme. According to Bergmann and Fruton (4), a cathepsin which is activated by either cysteine or ascorbic acid is classified as cathepsin III (also cf. 24). The synthetic substrate for cathepsin III is leucinamide. When leucinamide was added to brain homogenate it was found to protect against inhibition by the virus or iron salts.

The concentration of leucinamide required for protection is very high. Other amides, esters of amino acids as well as various peptides, were

TABLE IV

PROTECTIVE EFFECT OF PEPTIDES, AMIDES, AND ESTERS OF AMINO ACIDS ON GLYCOLYSIS OF BRAIN HOMOGENATES

	Compounds tested	Protective activity
Peptides	Glycylglycine, leucylglycine	Inactive
	Glycylleucine, glycylserine	Inactive
	Glycylasparagine	Inactive
	Leucylglycylglycylglycylglycine	Inactive
	D-Alanylglycine	Inactive
	Glutathione	Very active
Amides	Leucinamide	Active
	Benzoylargininamide	Weakly active
	Glutamine, asparagine	Inactive
	Malonamide	Weakly active
	Urea	Inactive
	Glycylleucinamide	Inactive
	Carbobenzoxyglycylleucinamide	Inactive
Esters	Leucine ethyl ester	Active
	Valine ethyl ester	Active
	Glycine ethyl ester	Active
	Glycylglycine ethyl ester	Active
	Cysteine ethyl ester	Active
	N-Phenylglycine ethyl ester	Very active

examined for protective activity. In Table IV a small fraction of the compounds tested is listed. Only the amide or ethyl ester of N-phenyl glycine proved to be considerably more effective than the amide or ester of leucine. We wish to thank Dr. Karl Pfister of the Merck Institute for his kindness in sending us various compounds which we tested in the hope that they might be more active than N-phenyglycyl ester. However, none of them were.

Let us briefly recapitulate the biochemical events as visualized (see Fig. 3) and explain the purpose of these experiments with amino-acid

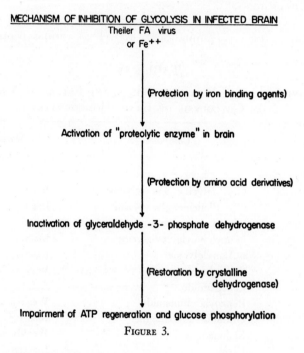

MECHANISM OF INHIBITION OF GLYCOLYSIS IN INFECTED BRAIN

Theiler FA virus
or Fe^{++}

(Protection by iron binding agents)

Activation of "proteolytic enzyme" in brain

(Protection by amino acid derivatives)

Inactivation of glyceraldehyde -3- phosphate dehydrogenase

(Restoration by crystalline dehydrogenase)

Impairment of ATP regeneration and glucose phosphorylation

FIGURE 3.

derivatives. We reasoned that the inhibition of triose phosphate dehydrogenase which we observed *in vitro* in the presence of the virus may actually occur *in vivo* and may be responsible for the cell destruction during infection. In this event a compound which protects triose phosphate dehydrogenase against the inactivation might help to preserve the neurons.

We failed to obtain a compound which would reach the brain in a concentration which might be expected to be effective. The esters and amides of amino acids tested by us are hydrolyzed in the animal body and do not readily penetrate the blood-brain barrier. We actually tried to deposit the phenyl glycine derivatives intracerebrally and the few animals who survived this gentle treatment seemed to be less susceptible to the encephalitis infection. But, for obvious reasons, we do not place much stock in these experiments.

Perhaps these studies should be resumed in tissue cultures to avoid the problem of the blood-brain barrier. The possibility that a similar defect of glucose metabolism operates in tissue cultures is suggested by the findings of Victor and Huang (25) and by the more recent studies of Enders and his collaborators (7) in connection with their diagnostic test for poliomyelitis viruses.

IV. CONCLUSIONS

Finally we may attempt to answer a question asked at the beginning. What can we learn from studies of the metabolism of infected cells?

The two studies chosen as examples in this discussion have yielded new information on specific features of host-cell metabolism. In the case of *E. coli,* new pathways of glucose-6-phosphate and ribose-5-phosphate utilization were explored, the biosynthesis of ribose-5-phosphate and desoxyribose-5-phosphate were studied, and interesting features of nucleic-acid metabolism and bacterial nutrition were revealed. In the study of brain metabolism information on the properties of several glycolytic enzymes were obtained. The significance of the observed alterations of the metabolism in relation to the infectious process remains, however, still in the realm of speculation.

In a discussion on the effect of chemotherapeutic agents on bacterial metabolism Dr. B. Davis once told the story of a drunkard. A drunkard has lost his key somewhere in the dark. But since he cannot see in the dark he searches for the key near the lamppost where he can see. I should like to give this story a new ending. The drunkard actually finds a key near the lamppost, but drunk as he is, he cannot tell whether it is his own. But just imagine the fine time he has sitting on the doorstep and dreaming about all the castles this key may open for him.

REFERENCES

1. Bauer, D. J. (1953). *in* The Nature of Virus Multiplication, p. 46. Cambridge University Press, England.
2. Bawden, F. C. (1950). Plant Viruses and Virus Diseases. Chronica Botanica, Waltham, Mass.
3. Berger, L., Slein, M. W., Colowick, S. P., and Cori, C. F. (1946). *J. Gen. Physiol.* 29, 379.
4. Bergmann, M., and Fruton, J. S. (1941). *Advances in Enzymol.* 1, 63.
5. Cohen, S. S. (1947). *Cold Spring Harbor Symposia Quant. Biol.* 12, 35.
6. Cohen, S. S. (1953). *Cold Spring Harbor Symposia Quant. Biol.* 18, 221.
7. Enders, J. F. (1952). *in* Poliomyelitis (The Second International Poliomyelitis Conference). J. B. Lippincott Co., Philadelphia.
8. Evans, Jr., E. A. (1952). Biochemical Studies of Bacterial Viruses. The University of Chicago Press, Chicago.
9. Hershey, A. D. (1953). *J. Gen. Physiol.* 37, 1.
10. Jacob, F. (1951). *Compt. rend.* 232, 1605.

11. Kozloff, L. M. (1953). *Cold Spring Harbor Symposia Quant. Biol.* 18, 209.
12. Krimsky, I. and Racker, E. (1949). *J. Biol. Chem.* 179, 903.
13. Lark, K. G. and Adams, M. H. (1953). *Cold Spring Harbor Symposia Quant. Biol.* 18, 171.
14. Lwoff, A. (1953). *in* The Nature of Virus Multiplication, p. 165. Cambridge University Press, England.
15. Racker, E. and Kabat, H. (1942). *J. Exptl. Med.* 76, 579.
16. Racker, E. and Krimsky, I. (1945). *J. Biol. Chem.* 161, 453.
17. Racker, E. and Krimsky, I. (1946). *J. Exptl. Med.* 84, 191.
18. Racker, E. and Krimsky, I. (1947). *J. Exptl. Med.* 85, 715.
19. Racker, E. (1947). *J. Biol. Chem.* 167, 843.
20. Racker, E. and Adams, M. H. (1947). *in* Annual Reports, p. 26. Long Island Biological Association, Cold Spring Harbor, N. Y.
21. Racker, E. and Krimsky, I. (1948). *J. Biol. Chem.* 173, 519.
22. Racker, E. (1948). *Federation Proc.* 7, 180.
23. Racker, E. (1952). *J. Biol. Chem.* 196, 347.
24. Tallan, H. H., Jones, M. E., and Fruton, J. S. (1952). *J. Biol. Chem.* 194, 793.
25. Victor, J. and Huang, C. H. (1944). *J. Exptl. Med.* 79, 129.
26. Wood, H. G., Rusoff, I. I., and Reiner, J. M. (1945). *J. Exptl. Med.* 81, 151.
27. Wood, H. G. and Utter, M. F. (1947). Personal communication.

A STUDY OF PHYTOPATHOGENIC MICROBIAL TOXINS OF KNOWN CHEMICAL STRUCTURE AND MODE OF ACTION

By D. W. Woolley, *The Rockefeller Institute for Medical Research, New York, N. Y.*

T HE FOLLOWING remarks are the result of a request to discuss Dr. Pappenheimer's paper, "Some Effects of Bacteria and Their Products on Host-cell Metabolism," page 102, by showing you briefly some examples we have uncovered. These findings indicate that in diseases of plants which are induced by certain microorganisms, the invading parasite produces a toxin. This toxin will reproduce the manifestations of the disease without the presence of the microorganism. The toxins which we have studied have been isolated in chemically pure form, and investigations of their chemical structures have revealed them to be small molecules, composed of a few amino acids. They have proved to be structural analogues of recognized essential compounds in the plant cells. In appropriate species, the toxins have been shown to antagonize the action of their structurally related cell constituents. These toxins are therefore antimetabolites which are produced by the microbial parasite and which damage the host tissue by causing a specific deficiency disease.

The first of these toxins to be so investigated was lycomarasmin. This phytopathogenic product of *Fusarium lycopersici* was first isolated in pure condition in 1944 by Plattner and Clauson-Kaas (1, 2). The fungus is the causative agent of a wilting disease of tomato plants. The isolated toxin will reproduce the signs of the disease, and, in fact, assays for it are performed by exposing excised tomato leaves to appropriate dilutions of the toxin, and noting the extent of the wilting and other typical changes which result in these tissues.

Our studies of the chemistry of lycomarasmin (3), in addition to the earlier work of Plattner and Clauson-Kaas (4), showed it to possess the structure shown on page 110. It is thus a rather unusual peptide composed of asparagine, glycine, and a new unstable amino acid, α-hydroxyalanine.

In tomato leaves, the toxic action of lycomarasmin is overcome by concentrates of the growth factor strepogenin (5). This growth factor is also a small peptide, and, so far as is known, is a derivative of glutamic acid with a few other amino acids. Its chemical structure is not completely known, but enough has been learned about it to recognize in it a resemblance to lycomarasmin. Although the structure of natural strepogenin has

149

not been completely established, a small peptide has been synthesized which has slight strepogenin activity both as a growth factor and as an antagonist to lycomarasmin. This peptide is serylglycylglutamic acid. This compound was synthesized as a result of the findings with lycomarasmin. It proved to be capable of overcoming the phytopathogenic properties of the toxin. Its structural resemblance to lycomarasmin is clear. A difficulty in the interpretation of these findings is that the antagonism between strepogenin and lycomarasmin is noncompetitive. Nevertheless, one can tentatively picture the wilting disease of tomatoes as being caused by, or at least related to, a strepogenin deficiency induced in the plant by this poisonous product of the invading fungus.

The second case which I want to mention is more recently investigated, and, in fact, is just now being completed. This is the case of the toxin of *Pseudomonas tabaci*. This bacterium invades tobacco and certain other farm crops, and causes wildfire disease. The trouble is so named because it sweeps through a field of tobacco like wildfire, causing clorotic spots to appear on the leaves. These lesions are due to a soluble toxin formed by the bacterium. This toxin, by itself, will reproduce the characteristic lesions

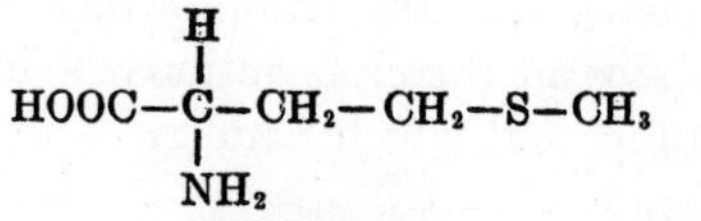

$$\underset{\substack{| \\ NH_2}}{HOOC-\overset{\overset{\displaystyle H}{|}}{C}-CH_2-CH_2-S-CH_3}$$

Methionine

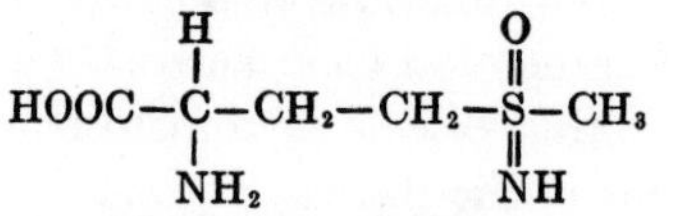

$$\underset{\substack{| \\ NH_2}}{HOOC-\overset{\overset{\displaystyle H}{|}}{C}-CH_2-CH_2-\underset{\substack{\| \\ NH}}{\overset{\displaystyle O}{\overset{\|}{S}}}-CH_3}$$

Methionine sulfoximine

$$\underset{\substack{| \\ NH_2}}{HOOC-\overset{\overset{\displaystyle H}{|}}{C}-CH_2-CH_2-\underset{\substack{| \\ H}}{\overset{\overset{\displaystyle HO}{|}}{C}}-\underset{\substack{| \\ NHCHO}}{\overset{\overset{\displaystyle H}{|}}{C}}-COOR}$$

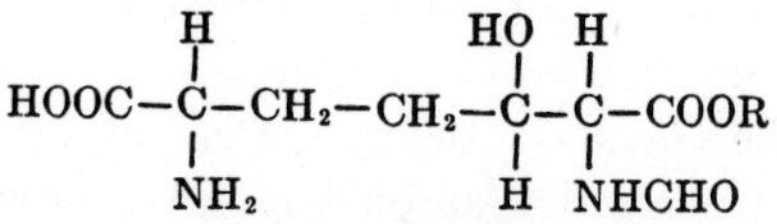

P. tabaci toxin

FIG. 1. STRUCTURES OF METHIONINE, METHIONINE SULFOXIMINE, AND THE TOXIN OF *P. tabaci*.

of the disease. The poisonous principle has recently been isolated in crystal-line form (6), and has proved to be a simple derivative of a new amino acid. Its structure has been established as that shown in Fig. 1. It is a very unstable substance which breaks down with great ease under various con-ditions to yield formic acid and the new amino acid. This latter compound, which is called tabtoxinine (7), is α,ε-diamino-β-hydroxypimelic acid. The only point still in doubt about the chemical structure of the toxin is the nature of the esterified alcohol, indicated by R in the slide. This is either a glycol of not more than three carbon atoms or else it is the alcoholic group of the tabtoxinine itself.

The work on this toxin of *P. tabaci* has been carried out in collaboration with Dr. A. C. Braun. He has shown that in certain species of plants, although not in tobacco, the poisonous action of this toxin can be reversed, in a competitive fashion, by methionine (8). No other substance capable of doing this has been found. The structure of methionine is shown on the slide, from which it is clear that the toxin and its naturally occurring antagonist are analogous. In fact, because of this antagonism the working hypothesis was formed that the toxin was probably an antimetabolite of methionine, and it was principally for this reason that the isolation and elucidation of the structure of the toxin were attempted. It has been gratifying to see the prediction come true.

The relationship of methionine and the toxin can be seen even more clearly in the following way: A synthetic antimetabolite of methionine was available. This was methionine sulfoximine which has recently been identified as the causative agent produced in wheat flour when it is bleached with nitrogen trichloride, and which is the causative agent of canine hysteria (9, 10, 11). This synthetic antimetabolite of methionine will cause the typical lesions in tobacco leaves which are elicited by the toxin of wildfire disease. If now we compare the structures of methionine, methionine sulfoximine, and the *Pseudomonas* toxin, the relationships will be quite evident. In the toxin the sulfur atom of the sulfoximine has been replaced by two carbon atoms, one of which bears the oxygen and the other the nitrogen atom originally attached to this sulfur. In addition, the oxygen and nitrogen bonds have been reduced, and the methyl group has been oxidized up to an ester grouping. One can regard the acylation of the nitrogen and the formation of an ester from the carboxyl as clever maneuvers of the bacterium to neutralize the electrical charge at the one end of the molecule so that the whole toxin would more closely resemble methionine.

Here then in the toxin of *P. tabaci* we find a second example of the production of an antimetabolite specifically directed against an important participating molecule in the cell of the host. Apparently, the invading parasite is able to cause damage in the tissues of the host by creation of a unique deficiency disease. In the plant kingdom these pathogenic toxins have, in the two instances cited, proved to be simple derivatives of amino acids. In the animal kingdom where, as we know, the microbial toxins have usually proved to be complex derivatives of amino acids, or in other words, proteins, we may yet find that the mechanism of action of these toxins is the same as that among plants. That is, the toxins may prove to be specific antimetabolites of important proteins in the cells of the animal host.

It has not been possible, in this brief discussion, to deal critically with many points. Nevertheless, it should be stated that all investigators are not in agreement on many of the things which have necessarily been stated categorically. It may even be that the major thesis will be challenged by some. Consequently, those who are interested in this subject are urged to read the rather extensive literature which has been published during the past 10 years.

REFERENCES

1. Plattner, P. A. and Clauson-Kaas, N. (1944). *Helv. Chim. Acta* 28, 188.
2. Clauson-Kaas, N., Plattner, P. A., and Gäumann, E. (1944). *Ber. schweiz. botan. Ges.* 54, 523.
3. Woolley, D. W. (1948). *J. Biol. Chem.* 176, 1291.
4. Plattner, P. A. and Clauson-Kaas, N. (1945). *Experientia* 1, 195.
5. Woolley, D. W. (1946). *J. Biol. Chem.* 166, 783.
6. Woolley, D. W., Pringle, R. B., and Braun, A. C. (1952). *J. Biol. Chem.* 197, 409.
7. Woolley, D. W., Schaffner, G., and Braun, A. C. (1952). *J. Biol. Chem.* 198, 807.
8. Braun, A. C. (1950). *Proc. Natl. Acad. Sci.* 36, 423.
9. Reiner, L., Misani, F., Fair, T. W., Weiss, P., and Cordasco, M. C. J. (1950). *J. Am. Chem. Soc.* 72, 2297.
10. Bentley, H. R., McDermott, E. E., Pace, J., Whitehead, J. K., and Moran, T. (1950). *Nature* 165, 150.
11. Campbell, P. N., Work, T. S., and Mellanby, E. (1951). *Biochem. J.* 48, 106.

INTRACELLULAR SURVIVAL OF BACTERIA IN ACUTE AND CHRONIC TUBERCULOSIS

By Hubert Bloch, *Division of Tuberculosis, The Public Health Research Institute of The City of New York, Inc., New York, N. Y.*

CHRONIC INFECTIONS, in contrast to acute infectious diseases, are an ill-defined entity. The term includes infections which after an acute initial stage fail to come to a quick end, persisting for a long time with little tendency for clinical change. Certain types of urinary or enteric bacterial infections or virus diseases such as infectious hepatitis may be quoted here. Under the same heading of chronic infections, there is another type of disease listed, the first clinical manifestations of which cannot be accurately related to the moment of infection. Pulmonary tuberculosis in man is the classical example of this category. Many years may elapse between the incidence of infection and the first appearance of clinical symptoms. Clearly, the infection as well as the disease are chronic by definition, but chronicity in this instance is less remarkable than the fact that the latent infection develops into a disease without an apparent time relationship between the two events. For all we know, infection, though necessary, is not sufficient for clinical tuberculosis to become manifest, because in the majority of cases tuberculous infection never leads to tuberculosis and the persistency of living tubercle bacilli capable of causing a specific disease does not, per se, give rise to tuberculosis. The bacillus and the host coexist within a kind of symbiosis which at any time and for a variety of causes may turn into a clinical disease. The kind of interrelationship between host cell and parasite which prevails in this system shall be the subject of the present discussion.

For all practical purposes, the tubercle bacillus in its natural occurrence is an intracellular parasite. Except for the special conditions of the caseum where the organism can undergo rapid multiplication (10) and its transitional appearance in the blood and in certain exudates, body cells are the natural habitat of the bacillus. After inhalation as well as following parenteral injection, the organism is phagocytized and henceforth survives intracellularly (15). There are no significant differences between the rate of phagocytosis of highly pathogenic bacteria and of organisms from attenuated or nonpathogenic strains (3). They all are rapidly engulfed

153

and thus taken out of circulation. From then on, their future state is determined by a variety of quite unrelated factors. These are: the inherent virulence of the strain, the physiological state of the bacterial suspension, the genetic susceptibility of the host species, the natural or acquired resistance of the individual host organism, and a number of so-called unspecific factors, such as hormonal regulations, nutrition, age, sex, and others.

In all instances where they cause disease, the bacilli multiply intracellularly. Multiplication depends on the factors just mentioned, often it is small and limited to a short period of time. But regardless of whether the mycobacteria multiply or not, they remain alive for long periods of time in the infected organism. Even bacteria from strains unable to multiply *in vivo* can be recovered for many weeks after they were injected into an animal. It may be recalled, though, that prolonged survival *in vivo* is not typical of the tubercle bacillus alone, but is true for many infectious agents, e.g. *Cl. tetani, C. diphtheriae,* the viruses of herpes, rabies, and others. In the case of mycobacteria, the resistance to being destroyed intracellularly may partly be due to their characteristic chemical structure because killed bacilli injected into an animal, too, remain detectable by staining techniques for a long time.

In man, living virulent bacilli are found in minimal tuberculous lesions of many healthy individuals not known to suffer from tuberculosis. In the organs where they are found, such bacilli hardly increase in numbers. They survive in a resting stage but under more favorable conditions, either in the test tube or in experimental animals, they start multiplying again.

The fact that the organisms survive indicates that they find adequate living conditions inside the host cell, but it fails to explain why, in many cases, bacteria of a pathogenic strain should not multiply in man or in an animal belonging to a species susceptible to progressive tuberculosis. Experiments designed to study this particular aspect of tuberculosis will be summarized shortly. The methods and techniques employed have been described in detail in various previous publications (5, 7).

Mice of an inbred strain (CFI), infected with a high dose (2×10^6 infectious units) of virulent tubercle bacilli (strain H37Rv), die within a narrow range of time (Fig. 1). Increasing the infective dose would shift the peak of this distribution to the left, but leave the general aspect of the curve unchanged.[1] If, however, a smaller infective dose is used, the curve not only shifts to the right, but it also changes its character (Fig. 2).

[1] The same would happen if a more virulent bacterial strain were chosen. It has been pointed out before that there is no way, in experimental tuberculosis, to distinguish an infection with a relatively small dose of highly virulent bacilli from the effects of a larger dose of organisms of lesser virulence (6).

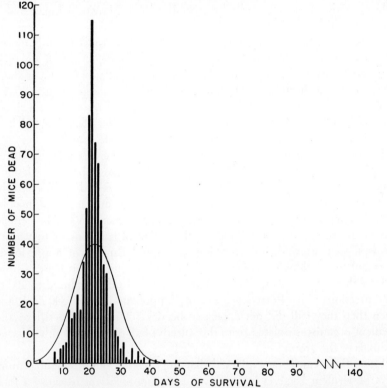

FIG. 1. HISTOGRAM SHOWING THE SURVIVAL TIMES OF 745 CFI MICE INFECTED INTRAVENOUSLY WITH 0.1 ML OF A 5-DAY TWEEN-ALBUMIN CULTURE OF H37Rv.

Median survival time, 20 days. All mice died of tuberculosis, 99.2% within 40 days after infection.

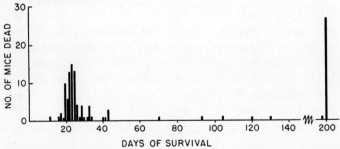

FIG. 2. HISTOGRAM SHOWING THE SURVIVAL OF 116 CFI MICE, INFECTED WITH 0.025 ML OF A 5-DAY CULTURE OF H37Rv.

Median survival time, 24 days. Ten mice (11%) died between 40 and 198 days. Twenty-seven mice (23%) were sacrificed 200 days after infection.

The deviation from the normal distribution curve shown in Fig. 2 makes it obvious that 4 to 5 weeks after infection the reaction of the mice to tuberculosis has changed. Since the animals used are from a highly inbred strain of mice, the shape of the curve cannot be the expression of a genetic inhomogeneity of the group. Similar survival curves flattening out at about 30 days after a sharp initial decline have been published previously (5, 16, 22). They are neither typical of a particular breed of mice nor of a single bacterial strain. Thus, they can only be the reflection of a changed host reaction, occurring during the first 30 days of the infection.

In the experiment summarized in Fig. 2, all survivors were sacrificed after 200 days. As was to be expected, they all had gross tuberculous lesions. Tubercle bacilli were easily cultured from their lungs and spleens and the cultures possessed the original virulence of the strain used for inoculation. The presence of virulent organisms in such mice can also be demonstrated by subjecting the animals to the action of cortisone or to various stresses, such as cold. The reaction is a rapid flare-up of a previously dormant tuberculous disease resulting in death within a short lapse of time.

In a third experiment, the infective dose was further reduced to 100 to 500 infectious units. Forty-seven out of 50 mice survived for 340 days, and even then they still did not appear to be sick.[2] They were sacrificed and virulent organisms isolated from the spleens of all of ten randomly selected animals of the group.

How, then, can it be explained that the presence of considerable numbers of virulent bacteria is, in many cases, not sufficient to cause a fatal disease provided the animal escaped death within the first 4 weeks after infection? Why is there a regular break in the survival curves one month after infection, instead of a steady decline?

A likely explanation is that in the course of infection the mice have acquired a degree of immunity protecting them for an extended period of time from the effects of the infection. The bacilli cease to multiply. Their prolonged survival in a resting, but inherently infective, state indicates that their multiplication is checked by an immune mechanism which the animal has acquired during the early phase of the infection. As time proceeds, the surviving organisms may continue to produce those antigens which are responsible for the lasting resistance in these animals. This inference makes the assumption that immunity can be produced by non-multiplying bacteria. To investigate the likelihood of this assumption, the

[2] It is noteworthy to point out in this connection that none of the often-quoted experimental single-cell infections in guinea pigs caused generalized fatal tuberculosis. In all instances, the animals were sacrificed, often after many months of observation (12, 21, 23).

reaction of mice to infection was tested after vaccination with nonpathogenic, nonmultiplying bacteria, and compared to the effects of vaccination with freely multiplying attenuated organisms. Strains of both varieties are available. Bacteria of the BCG strain multiply in mice, whereas organisms of the strain H37Ra fail to do so (20). This provides the opportunity to compare the degree of protection achieved with multiplying and nonmultiplying organisms.

It has been found in numerous experiments in mice as well as in guinea pigs that living bacilli of the nonmultiplying strain H37Ra are as good, if not better vaccines than equal numbers of multiplying BCG (17). Further information on the role of bacterial multiplication during vaccination was obtained from experiments where increase in numbers of BCG was arrested by high doses of isoniazid administered throughout the vaccination period. Bacterial counts and control experiments with virulent bacilli have shown that under these conditions isoniazid is highly effective in arresting bacterial multiplication.[3] Despite this, the degree of protection afforded was the same as with freely multiplying BCG vaccine (Table I). Thus, in the mouse, the effectiveness of a vaccine depends on bacterial survival rather than on bacterial multiplication. There is no contradiction in the fact that immunity was conferred by resting pathogenic organisms in one instance, and by nonmultiplying, nonpathogenic bacilli in the other, because we do not know of antigenic differences *with regard to immunity* between virulent and nonvirulent tubercle bacilli.

However, it is essential that the vaccine contains viable bacilli. The immunity resulting from bacterial preparations killed by various techniques (heat, phenol, irradiation), or from injections of various bacterial extracts, was poor as compared to the one produced by living organisms (17).

The assumption does not seem unreasonable that mice surviving for very extended periods of time after being infected with large doses of virulent organisms owe their relative immunity to the living tubercle bacilli they harbor in their organs. Likewise, the immunity found in tuberculin-positive, nontuberculous human individuals appears to be of the same kind. In each of these instances there is a common feature, i.e., bacilli surviving intracellularly for long periods of time without causing clinical tuberculosis. This status which may remain stationary during the lifetime of an individual bears many of the characteristics of true commensalism (11). In the host cell, the microorganisms find living conditions suitable for survival, but their reproduction is closely checked by the host and the

---

[3] While isoniazid interferes most effectively with bacterial multiplication, it does not eradicate the bacilli completely. Numerous organisms survive intracellularly.

TABLE I

THE INFLUENCE OF ISONIAZID[a] ON THE EFFECT OF BCG VACCINATION
IN MICE

Group No.[b]	Prechallenge treatment	Total vaccina- tion period (days)	No. of survivors 80 days after challenge[d]	Median survival time (days)
1	3 days after vaccination,[c] isoniazid treatment was started and continued for 14 days	17	15/20	> 80
2	Vaccinated the same day on which isoniazid was started and treatment continued for 14 days	14	12/20	> 80
3	BCG control I: vaccinated 17 days before challenge	17	15/20	> 80
4	BCG control II: vaccinated 3 days before challenge	3	2/20	23
5	Infection control I: these mice were given isoniazid for 14 days before they were challenged	— —	1/20	24
6	Infection control II: no prechallenge treat-ment	— —	2/20	23

[a]Isoniazid was given as a 0.1% addition to powdered pellets. The daily intake was about 4 mg per mouse. The mice were challenged the same day on which isoniazid treatment was discontinued. The experiment was organized in such a way that all groups were challenged at the same time and with the same bacterial culture.

[b]20 mice per group.

[c]All mice were vaccinated with 0.075 mg (wet weight) BCG.

[d]All survivors were sacrificed after 80 days.

bacilli are limited to certain areas. Paradoxically, in this case the factors which control multiplication of the infecting bacilli have been specifically activated by these very same bacilli.

At this stage, bacterium and host organism are in a delicate state of equilibrium which is subject to being disturbed by a number of different impacts. For obvious reasons, it is easy to observe actions resulting in an activiation of the hitherto dormant infection, whereas an increase in resistance followed by complete eradication of the bacilli is technically difficult, if not impossible, to demonstrate. Activation of the infection can be caused by specific as well as nonspecific influences. The best documented example of the latter group is the enhancing action which cortisone exerts on chronic tuberculosis. This effect is nonspecific. Tuberculosis is but one of many unrelated infections aggravated by injections of this hormone.

On the other hand, a similar activation and enhancement of experimental tuberculosis may be brought about by injections of small amounts of "cord factor," a toxic lipid-carbohydrate-nitrogen complex obtained from virulent tubercle bacilli (4, 18), or by supplementing a relatively small infective dose with injections of small amounts of "cord factor" (Table II).

TABLE II

THE EFFECT OF A SINGLE INJECTION OF 0.01 MG CORD FACTOR, DISSOLVED IN 0.1 ML PARAFFIN OIL, FOLLOWED 24 HOURS LATER BY INTRAVENOUS INFECTION WITH VARIOUS DILUTIONS OF A 6-DAY CULTURE OF H37RV (UNDILUTED INOCULUM: APPROX. 5×10^6 INFECTIOUS UNITS)

No. of mice per group	Amount of cord factor injected (mg)	Infective dose	Individual survival times (days after infection)[a]
10	0.01	1 : 1	11, 13, 17, 18, 19, 20, 21, 21, 21, 22
10	0.01	1 : 2	11, 14, 14, 20, 22, 23, 24, 28, 29, 30
10	0.01	none	S, S, S, S, S, S, S, S, S, S
10	none[b]	1 : 1	20, 22, 24, 35, 38, S, S, S, S, S
10	none	1 : 2	20, 23, 23, 25, 27, S, S, S, S, S

[a]The animals marked with S were sacrificed 50 days after infection when the experiment was discontinued.

[b]The infection control animals received an injection of 0.1 ml bayol (light paraffin oil).

Cord factor is produced and secreted by strains of tubercle bacilli able to multiply in a susceptible host (1). It is not found in organisms of avirulent strains, such as H37Ra (4, 19). In vitro, it is synthesized more abundantly by rapidly multiplying, young cultures than by older ones (8). Likewise, it has been shown that young cultures are considerably more virulent than equal numbers of viable bacteria from older cultures (4, 13). The production of cord factor by the bacterial cell can be specifically inhibited in vitro without, at the same time, inhibiting bacterial growth (7). Some compounds having this action are active antituberculous chemotherapeutics. As such, however, they merely arrest bacterial multiplication and their effect ceases to be noticeable after discontinuation of the drug.

On the basis of these observations, it is suggested that cord factor, by being released by the bacillus into the surrounding menstruum, specifically causes the type of injury to the host cell which creates favorable conditions for bacterial multiplication. In this sense, it may function as an "aggressin" (?, 14). In contrast to cortisone, the action of cord factor is specific. None of a variety of bacterial and virus infections is influenced by doses which greatly enhance the severity of both acute and chronic tuberculous infections (9). Nevertheless, it is likely that both specific and nonspecific factors act by making intracellular conditions more favorable for bacterial multiplication, rather than by directly stimulating the bacterial growth and multiplication. None of the agents mentioned has visible effects on bacterial cultures *in vitro*.

During the chronic phase, the tuberculous infection remains stationary. Despite the continuous presence of living infectious organisms, clinical signs of tuberculosis are lacking. The animal (or man) has acquired a considerable degree of immunity against new infections, but at the same time he is liable to an exacerbation of his own condition after having been exposed to a variety of seemingly unrelated impacts such as stress, nutritional or endocrine changes, or intecurrent infections other than tuberculosis. There is no doubt that a great majority of the hospital cases of human tuberculosis owe their immediate origin to such nonspecific impacts and that the incidence of the specific infection represents merely the necessary premise to the event. On the other hand, the presence of live bacilli indirectly responsible for the outbreak of tuberculosis will protect the individual in other instances from the consequences of massive new tuberculous infection.

Teleologically speaking, the harboring of resting tubercle bacilli is a double-edged sword and there is as yet no decision in the treatment of tuberculosis as to whether eradicating tubercle bacilli completely is a desirable therapeutic goal or not. The answer cannot come from taking into consideration the individual case alone. It has to be formed upon the evaluation of the over-all epidemiological picture as well as by evaluating the chances of an individual being exposed to a new infection in the surroundings in which he lives. In many cases, it might well be possible to use specific vaccination as an adjunct to the present methods of surgery and chemotherapy in the treatment of tuberculosis.

REFERENCES

1. Asselineau, J., Bloch, H., and Lederer, E. (1953). *Am. Rev. Tuberc.* 67, 853.
2. Bail, O., and Weil, E. (1911). *Arch. Hyg.* 73, 218.
3. Bloch, H. (1948). *Am. Rev. Tuberc.* 68, 662.

4. Bloch, H. (1950). *J. Exptl. Med.* 91, 197.
5. Bloch, H. (1950). *J. Exptl. Med.* 92, 507.
6. Bloch, H. (1953). *Ann. Rev. Microbiol.* 8, 19.
7. Bloch, H., and Noll, H. (1953). *J. Exptl. Med.* 97, 1.
8. Bloch, H., Sorkin, E., and Erlenmeyer, H. (1953). *Am. Rev. Tuberc.* 67, 629.
9. Bloch, H. Unpublished observation.
10. Canetti, G. (1946). Le bacille de Koch dans la lésion tuberculeuse du poumon. Paris.
11. Caullery, M. (1950). Le parasitisme et la symbiose. Paris.
12. Doerr, R., and Gold, E. (1932). *Z. Immunitätsforsch.* 74, 7.
13. Fenner, F., and Leach, R. H. (1953). *Am. Rev. Tuberc.* 68, 321.
14. Keppie, J., Smith, H., and Harris-Smith, P. W. (1953). *Brit. J. Exptl. Pathol.* 34, 486.
15. Lurie, M. B. (1950). *Am. J. Med.* 9, 591.
16. McKee, C. M., Rake, G., Donovick, R., and Jambor, W. P. (1949). *Am. Rev. Tuberc.* 60, 90.
17. Nissen-Meyer, S., Palmer, C. E., Segal, W., and Bloch, H. To be published.
18. Noll, H., and Bloch, H. (1953). *Am. Rev. Tuberc.* 67, 828.
19. Noll, H., Lederer, E., and Bloch, H. To be published.
20. Pierce, C. H., Dubos, R. J., and Schaefer, W. B. (1953). *J. Exptl. Med.* 97, 189.
21. Schwabacher, H., and Wilson, G. S. (1937). *Tubercle* 18, 442.
22. Svedberg, B. (1951). *Acta Med. Scand.* 139, *Suppl.,* 254.
23. Wämoscher, L., and Stoecklin, K. (1927). *Zentr. Bakteriol. Parasitenk., Abt. I (Orig.)* 104, 86.

INHIBITION OF THEILER'S GDVII VIRUS BY AN INTESTINAL MUCOPOLYSACCHARIDE

By Benjamin Mandel, *Division of Infectious Diseases, The Public Health Research Institute of the City of New York*

Dr. Adams has discussed the role of polysaccharides in certain viral infections. Under the same heading I should like to describe the relationship of a mucopolysaccharide to another viral disease, murine encephalomyelitis. This disease is caused by Theiler's virus (1, 2) of which there are several strains, e.g., TO and GDVII. The TO strain is present in the intestinal tract of almost all adult laboratory mice but causes no clinically manifest infection (3). However, in rare instances this virus invades the central nervous system and produces a poliomyelitis-like disease. The same disease follows the artificial introduction of TO virus by intracerebral inoculation. GDVII is pathogenic by the intracerebral route but in contrast to TO is not known to occur in the intestinal tract.

The present discussion is concerned mainly with the inhibition of the GDVII strain, a hemagglutinating as well as neurotropic agent, by a mucopolysaccharide (4, 5). This inhibitor is obtained from the intestinal tissue of adult mice and is purified from tissue extracts by removal of lipids and proteins and precipitation of the polysaccharide with ethanol. The purified inhibitor consists of about 50% reducing sugars, 30% hexosamine, and smaller quantities of galactose, hexuronic acid, and methylpentose. Several amino acids are liberated on acid hydrolysis. By means of chromatographic analysis it has been shown that the carbohydrate and amino acid components migrated in a closely parallel manner and their distribution coincided with the distribution of the biologically active material. It has therefore been inferred that the inhibitor is a polysaccharide-amino acid complex.

In vitro as little as 0.0002 µg of the most active preparations inhibits one unit of hemagglutinin. *In vivo* quantitation is less precise but it can be shown that about 0.0005 µg neutralizes one LD_{50} of virus.

Inhibition of viral activity is the result of interaction of virus and mucopolysaccharide with the formation of an inactive complex. Treatment of this complex with an enzyme results in the restoration of infectivity and hemagglutinin. This enzyme is obtained from the feces of mice where it is produced by a species of enteric bacterium.

162

Studies on the distribution of the inhibitor have shown that it is present in significant quantity in the stomach as well as the small intestine of adult mice, but not in other organs. Although it is present in the small intestine of infant mice, the quantity is considerably less than that found in adult animals. Small intestine of guinea pig, but not of other species which were tested, contains inhibitor.

The activity of this inhibitor seems to be highly specific. The FA and TO strains of Theiler's virus and the mouse-adapted Lansing strain of poliomyelitis virus are not affected.

Inhibition of GDVII virus is an example of neutralization by a non-immunological substance derived from the very host for which the virus is pathogenic. Of interest are the observations that in adult mice TO virus is present, and presumably multiplying, in the tissue from which the inhibitor is obtained, whereas in infant mice the same tissue is consistently free of TO virus and contains a considerably lesser quantity of inhibitor. What might be the implications of these findings? Dr. Adams has described certain polysaccharides, or receptor substances, and their role in mediating the union between virus and host cell. If we extend this concept to the Theiler viruses, it seems possible on purely speculative grounds that the mucopolysaccharide found in the intestine is the receptor substance for the TO virus and that it may be chemically and physically similar to the receptor substance of GDVII virus. As a result of this similarity, GDVII is able to react with the mucopolysaccharide but the reaction product is not reversible as would be the case for the homologous receptor substance.

Of interest also is the possibility that GDVII could multiply in the intestinal tract were it not for the presence of the inhibitor. Should this be true, the production of the mucopolysaccharide by the intestine would represent a nonimmunological protective mechanism of a tissue against an infectious agent.

REFERENCES

1. Theiler, M. (1937). *J. Exptl. Med.* 65, 705.
2. Theiler, M. and Gard, S. (1940). *J. Exptl. Med.* 72, 49.
3. Olitsky, P. K. (1939). *Proc. Soc. Exptl. Biol. Med.* 41, 434.
4. Mandel, B. and Racker, E. (1953). *J. Exptl. Med.* 98, 399.
5. Mandel, B. and Racker, E. (1953). *J. Exptl. Med.* 98, 417.

RELATION OF AN ENZYME DEPHOSPHORYLATING ADENOSINE TRIPHOSPHATE TO THE VIRUS OF AVIAN ERYTHROMYELOBLASTIC LEUKOSIS

By J. W. Beard, *Department of Surgery, Duke University School of Medicine, Durham, North Carolina*

It seems appropriate to the purpose of the symposium to relate briefly the results of recent work implicating a virus as the source of an enzyme dephosphorylating adenosine triphosphate. This virus is the etiological agent of erythromyeloblastosis, which is the leukemic form of the avian leukosis complex (1). One of the first members of the group of virus-induced tumors to be described (2), the condition is a highly malignant disease characterized by the occurrence in the circulation of large numbers of primitive white blood cells of erythroblastic or myeloblastic derivation. The viral etiology of erythromyeloblastic leukosis has been repeatedly verified, and the occurrence of the virus in the blood plasma of chicks with the disease has been unequivocally established.

Despite the considerable knowledge of the pathology and other aspects of the disease, little was known of the virus until recently. In 1949, there was undertaken a systematic study of this virus tumor directed principally toward investigation of the nature of the causative agent. Experiments involving ultracentrifugation of the plasma from diseased birds revealed a particulate material (3) of characteristic morphology (4) as disclosed in electron micrographs. The absence of similar particles in normal plasmas and the apparently specific relation of the particles to the disease, in which they occur in amounts reaching levels as high as 2×10^{12} particles per milliliter of plasma, stimulated the natural conclusion that the particles were identical with the virus. Disruption of the simplicity of this concept occurred in 1952 with the observation (5) that the plasmas from the diseased chickens were extremely active *in vitro* in the dephosphorylation of adenosine triphosphate. Especially confusing was the finding that this property was also associated with a material concentrated by ultracentrifugation in those fractions containing the particles presumed to represent the virus. It was possible, still, to suspect that the particles possessed an intrinsic constituent exerting the enzymatic activity. Alternative to this possibility was the existence of two populations of particles either indistinguishable in the electron microscope or in such relative numbers that one population, the virus particles or the enzyme particles, failed to attain the concentration necessary for demonstration by electron micrography. It was also possible that the particles might be the virus onto which the enzyme was adsorbed.

With the problem in this uncertain state, it became imperative to attempt, quantitatively, to establish the interrelationship, or lack of it, between the three plasma attributes. This was undertaken in a study of the relationship (*a*) as it developed with onset of the disease; (*b*) on electrophoresis of plasma; and (*c*) on ultracentrifugation of plasma. Particle concentration was estimated by direct counts (6, 7) of the particles sedimented on agar and taken off in a collodion film for electron micrography. Enzyme activity was determined by electrometric titration (7, 8) of the acid formed in the hydrolysis of adenosine triphosphate, and the infectious capacities of the plasmas were measured on the basis of latent-period procedures devised (9, 10) for application to the characters of host response to the erythromyelobastic leukosis virus. The plasmas were obtained from White Leghorn chicks (10, 11) of Line 15 (Regional Poultry Research Laboratory, East Lansing, Michigan) and injected intravenously at 3 days of age with 0.1 ml inoculums of previous passage plasma. The age of the birds at the time of bleeding varied from 19 to 80 days. Birds were selected as donors of the plasmas on the basis of a micro test (8, 12) for enzyme activity from the population exhibiting the disease diagnosed by routine blood smears. All of the plasmas, prevented from clotting by heparin, were filtered through celite and Selas bacteriological filters.

The experiments revealed (7) a very close correlation between the number of the specific particles and the enzyme activity of the plasmas. This was especially the case with the plasmas of higher particle content with which the counting technique yielded the most accurate estimates. The findings extended through the range of 5×10^9 to 859×10^9 particles per milliliter. Studies on electrophoretic behavior (13) revealed identical mobilities of the particles and the enzyme-bearing material in the pH region of 6.0 to 8.5. In the sedimentation experiments (13, 14), the particles were thrown down at the rate of $645s$, not significantly different from that observed with the enzyme, $597s$. The results of the titration were less decisive, but there was clearly a linear relation between virus infectivity and both particles and enzyme in the plasmas with onset of the disease. In the electrophoresis experiments, the virus moved at essentially the same rate as the enzyme and the particles. The sedimentation rate of the virus was $700s$, a value similar to the values found with the particles and the enzyme.

These experiments have shown that the virus, the particles, and the enzyme occur with quantitative simultaneity in the plasma with the development of the disease in injected birds. Furthermore, the three attributes are inseparable by electrophoresis or by sedimentation. Though the results do not provide unequivocal proof of the identity of the virus and enzyme with the single demonstrable population of specific particles, they do constitute strong evidence against the existence of two different kinds of particles. It is natural to suspect that the enzyme might be associated with particulate cellular elements deposited in the plasma on degradation of cellular elements. That extensive breakdown of cells is likely is indicated by the high plasma content of the ordinarily intracellular elements potassium and magnesium (15). These elements may have been derived through destruction of the red cells since anemia develops rapidly with onset of the disease. There is, at present, no indication of considerable breakdown of primitive cells, though degradation even of these cells would be expected to be conducive to liberation of virus as of cellular elements. No evidence has been seen in electron micrographs of more than one kind of particle, and the existence of two populations of particles occurring simultaneously and with closely similar electrophoretic and sedimentation properties is remote.

Investigation has shown (16) that the properties of the material dephosphorylating adenosine triphosphate are those of an enzyme. The enzyme is activated somewhat by Na^+ and K^+, acting separately or together and in a similar way by Ca^{++} and Mg^{++}, separately or in mixtures of the two. A very strong activating influence is seen, however, with either or both Ca^{++} and Mg^{++} in the presence of either or both monovalent ions. The concentrations of the ions optimum for the effects in a mixture of all were Na^+ and K^+, 0.05 M; and Ca^{++} and Mg^{++}, 0.04 M. The activating influence of the ions can be extinguished by chelation of the divalent ions. There is a strong dependence of the activity on hydrogen-ion concentration with a sharp single optimum at pH 7.16. Dephosphorylation involves hydrolysis only of the terminal phosphate of adenosine triphosphate, there being no effect on adenosine diphosphate either by hydrolysis or dismutation. Adenylic acid, which was not a reaction product and which was investigated separately, was not affected.

It would appear that the interpretations most closely compatible with the data indicate an intimate association of the particles, the virus and the enzyme. The principal question, then, is the nature of the association, i.e., whether the enzyme is adsorbed onto the virus particle or whether it is an intrinsic part of it. The possible association of enzymes with viruses has been the subject of much consideration, and, since access to purified viruses in 1934, has been put to experimental test in many investigations, particularly with the influenza virus. The results of the studies with the influenza virus occupy, in some respects, a special category. Here the specificity of the virus in its adsorption on and elution from red blood cells associates the virus unequivocally with the mechanism responsible for the phenomenon, and there has been little question (17) of the hypothesis that a mucinase is a constituent of the agent. In contrast the status of the problem with the virus of erythromyeloblastic leukosis is somewhat similar to the questions of the relation of certain enzymes, principally phosphatases, to bacteriophage (18) and to the virus of vaccinia (19–21) where the presence of enzymes is demonstrable, but the relation to the agents has been questioned.

It would be fruitless, at the present stage of the investigation, to insist that the dephosphorylating enzyme is a natural biological constituent of the virus of erythromyeloblastic leukosis rather than an adsorbed material. Certain facts, however, must be taken into account. If the phenomenon is related to adsorption, the adsorbed material must be of low molecular weight since it is plain that no material which might have the sedimentation properties of the specific particles can be seen attached to the particules. Furthermore, there is no evidence of a low-molecular-weight material with the enzyme properties in either normal or diseased plasmas. Thus, adsorption, if it occurs, must take place within the host cell by the incorporation within the surface of the virus of material sufficiently small in size as to be indiscernible by electron micrography. In addition the extent of adsorption on individual, different particles must occur with quantitative proportionality since enzyme activity is so closely related to particle count, not only in a given chick host but from one host to another. Biologically the enzyme exhibits a specific behavior quantitatively no different from that expected of an intrinsically incorporated constituent. In this respect the nature of the relationship is indistinguishable from that of analogous enzymes occurring with myosin and with cellular particulate components or of the mucinase activity with influenza virus.

Any consideration of the biological significance of the enzyme activity associated with the erythromyeloblastic leukosis virus must be entirely speculative. Adenosine triphosphate is a principal source of energy (22) widely distributed and involved in tissue metabolism. If, as it appears to be, the adenosine triphosphatase is a part of or firmly bound to the virus particle, there is no reason to suppose that the quality is lost in the process of entering the host cell. Under these conditions it is possible that the virus might exercise *in vivo* the enzyme activity demonstrable *in vitro*.

Per se, this would consist only in hydrolysis of the terminal phosphate of the substrate, a useless reaction and one possibly detrimental to both cellular and viral metabolism and synthesis unless there existed the requisite mechanism for energy transfer and utilization. However, in every instance adequately investigated, it has been evident that adenosine triphosphatase activity has been associated with energy transfer. There is, therefore, no reason to regard simple hydrolysis as the sole capacity of the adenosine triphosphatase associated with the leukosis virus. Various concepts have been proposed to account for the mechanism of virus increase within the cell, all involving various aspects of, thus far, undemonstrable enzymatic activities. Many theoretical aspects of a plausible energy spectrum needed for the processes might be postulated, including the activity of redirected adenosine triphosphatase in the initiation of steps toward energy utilization. In addition it is necessary to postulate the requisite specific substrates and coenzymes involved in completion of energy transfer. It is possible that the enzyme of the leukosis virus constitutes the first experimentally demonstrable significant link in the chain of enzyme materials necessary for the metabolism of the particular agent. There is some experimental evidence for the essentiality of high-energy phosphate bonds in the synthesis of some viruses in the observation, for example, of the suppression of influenza virus multiplication (23) in the presence of dinitrophenol. In addition to considerations relative to the leukosis virus, the possible interference of the virus enzyme in the metabolic function of the host cell with resultant effects influencing transformation of the normal to the malignant state should not be overlooked.

The present findings with the leukosis virus emphasize the need for reconsideration of the earlier experiments with bacteriophage and those of Macfarlane and her coworkers and of Hoagland et al. with vaccinia virus. The possibility that virus particles are able to adsorb enzyme should not constitute evidence that the particles may not already possess an intrinsic enzyme component. The thesis of pessimism and doubt of past accomplishments constitutes no acceptable deterrent to further investigations in this field.

REFERENCES

1. Jungherr, E., Dobyle, L. P., and Johnson, E. P. (1941). *Am. J. Vet. Research* 2, 116.
2. Ellermann, V. (1921). Leucosis of Fowls and Leucemia Problems. Gyldendal, London.
3. Beard, D., Eckert, E. A., Csáky, T. Z., Sharp, D. G., and Beard, J. W. (1950). *Proc. Soc. Exptl. Biol. Med.* 75, 533.
4. Sharp, D. G., Eckert, E. A., Beard, D., and Beard, J. W. (1952). *J. Bacteriol.* 63, 151.

5. Mommaerts, E. B., Eckert, E. A., Beard, D., and Beard, J. W. (1952). *Proc. Soc. Exptl. Biol. Med.* 79, 450.

6. Sharp, D. G. and Beard, J. W. (1952). *Proc. Soc. Exptl. Biol. Med.* 81, 75.

7. Mommaerts, E. B., Sharp, D. G., Eckert, E. A., Beard, D., and Beard, J. W. *J. Natl. Cancer Inst.* 14, 1011.

8. Green, I., Beard, D., Eckert, E. A., and Beard, J. W. *Proc. Soc. Exptl. Biol Med.* In press.

9. Eckert, E. A., Beard, D., and Beard, J. W. (1951). *J. Natl. Cancer Inst.* 12, 447.

10. Eckert, E. A., Beard, D., and Beard, J. W. *J. Natl. Cancer Inst.* 14, 1055.

11. Eckert, E. A., Waters, N. F., Burmester, B. R., Beard, D., and Beard, J. W. *J. Natl. Cancer Inst.* 14, 1067.

12. Mommaerts, E. B., Beard, D., and Beard, J. W. (1953). *Proc. Soc. Exptl. Biol. Med.* 83, 479.

13. Sharp, D. G., Mommaerts, E. B., Eckert, E. A., Beard, D., and Beard, J. W. *J. Natl. Cancer Inst.* 14, 1027.

14. Sharp, D. G., and Beard, J. W. *Biochim. et Biophys. Acta.* 14, 12.

15. Green, I., Beard, D., and Beard, J. W. In preparation.

16. Green, I., Beard, D., and Beard, J. W. In preparation.

17. Bauer, D. J. (1953). *in* The Nature of Virus Multiplication, pp. 46–84. Cambridge University Press, England.

18. Schüler, H. (1935). *Biochem. Z.* 276, 254.

19. Macfarlane, M. G. and Salaman, M. H. (1938). *Brit. J. Exptl. Pathol.* 19, 184.

20. Macfarlane, M. G. and Dolby, D. E. (1940). *Brit. J. Exptl. Pathol.* 21, 219.

21. Hoagland, C. L., Ward, S. M., Smadel, J. E., and Rivers, T. M. (1942). *J. Exptl. Med.* 76, 168.

22. Lipmann, F. (1941). *Advances in Enzymol.* 1, 99.

23. Ingraham, J. L., Roby, T. O., and Peterson, J. H. (1953). *Arch. Biochem. and Biophys.* 46, 215.

ALTERATION OF HOST ENERGY METABOLISM DURING INFECTION

By GIFFORD B. PINCHOT, *Department of Microbiology, Yale University School of Medicine, New Haven, Connecticut*

W E FIRST BECAME INTERESTED in the effects produced by infectious diseases on host-energy metabolism while studying tularemia in rats. This infection produced a profound fall in body temperature—sometimes reaching 14 to 15 Fahrenheit degrees below normal—which lasted several hours before the animals died. A similar hypothermia was observed after injecting large numbers of living *E. coli* cells intravenously (1). This observation suggested a marked interference with the infected animals' ability to produce energy. Accordingly, Dr. Walter L. Bloom and I set out to investigate the problem from this point of view. We found that diphtheria toxin also lowered the temperature of animals injected with it, we then used this toxin because it had the obvious advantages over active infections of being easier to work with and of giving more reproducible results.

We found that the injection of diphtheria toxin caused a 40% fall in the level of muscle phosphocreatine in guinea pigs, although the adenosine triphosphate levels remained unchanged. While this change does not seem very dramatic, it should be remembered that it occurred in resting muscles where the utilization of energy-rich phosphorus compounds was at a minimum. The reduction in high energy phosphate reserves presumably represents, therefore, a reduction in the rate at which these compounds are being formed in the intoxicated muscles. Arterial and venous oxygen studies were carried out to see if these changes were the results of peripheral circulatory collapse, but there was no evidence that the changes in phosphocreatine level could be explained by inadequate oxygen transport to the tissues (2).

It seemed reasonable to suppose, therefore, that the toxin had somehow interfered with the coupling of phosphorylation to oxidation. This aspect of the problem was studied with Dr. E. Racker, who was then at New York University. We found that pigeon-breast muscle, into which diphtheria toxin had been injected, had a much lower P/O ratio than the control muscle from the other side of the same bird. These results were

170

open to the criticism that the toxin might have caused a local and non-specific damage in the muscle, and the next step was to see if similar changes occurred in the heart following injection of the toxin into the pectoral muscle. Here again we found that the P/O ratios in heart-muscle homogenates from the intoxicated birds were lower than in the controls in each day's experiment, but over a period of weeks the control and experimental groups showed such marked variations that there was overlap between the results from the two groups. We felt that it would be more profitable to come back to this problem when more knowledge of the mechanisms of oxidative phosphorylation was available. It should be pointed out, however, that a defect in oxidative phosphorylation would fit very well with Dr. Pappenheimer's work indicating that diphtheria toxin acts by blocking synthesis of one of the cytochromes in the host, since a decrease in cytochrome would be expected to have an adverse effect on oxidative phosphorylation.

Dr. Racker and I then turned to a study of oxidative phosphorylation in pigeon-breast muscle and later in extracts of *E. coli*. In the bacterial extracts we found we could demonstrate inorganic phosphate esterification during alcohol oxidation, and that there were at least two components involved in the reaction which could be separated by means of ammonium sulfate and high-speed centrifugation. One fraction catalyzed the oxidation of reduced diphosphopyridine nucleotide (DPNH) formed by the alcohol dehydrogenase reaction, but it did this without phosphorylation. The second component restored phosphorylation when added to the oxidase fraction (3, 4).

The *E. coli* extracts catalyzed glycolysis and other phosphorylating reactions, however, which had to be prevented with inhibitors, and it was felt that the use of these inhibitors might have an adverse effect on phosphorylation coupled to electron transport. A bacterial system was looked for which would not have this disadvantage, and *Alcaligenes faecalis* extracts proved highly suitable, since they carried out phosphorylation associated with oxidation of alcohol or preformed reduced DPN, without any of the confusing side reactions. Here again it was possible to divide the extracts into two fractions, one of which catalyzed DPNH oxidation without phosphorylation, and the second of which restored the phosphorylation (5). It has also recently been possible to separate these fractions by centrifugation at $105,000 \times g$. The DPNH oxidase is precipitated and the phosphorylating component remains in the supernatant solution. The amount of phosphorylation observed is proportional to the amount of phosphorylating component added, and this fraction is now being purified.

It is of some interest perhaps in connection with the discussion of the unity or disunity in biochemistry that oxidative phosphorylation in extracts of *E. coli* and *Alcaligenes faecalis* is not affected by concentrations of 2,4 dinitrophenol which completely inhibit this reaction in animal mitochondria, and that levels of sodium fluoride, which have been used to increase ATP in animal mitochondria by inhibiting ATPase, are strongly inhibitory to phosphorylation associated with electron transport in the *Alcaligenes faecalis* extracts.

REFERENCES

1. Pinchot, G. B., Close, V. P., and Long, C. N. H. (1949). *Endocrinology* 45, 135.
2. Pinchot, G. B. and Bloom, W. L. (1950). *J. Biol. Chem.* 184, 9.
3. Pinchot, G. B. and Racker, E. (1951). *Federation Proc.* 10, 233.
4. Pinchot, G. B. and Racker, E. (1950). *in* Phosphorus Metabolism, ed. by W. D. McElroy and B. Glass, Vol. 1, p. 366. The Johns Hopkins Press, Baltimore.
5. Pinchot, G. B. (1953). *J. Biol. Chem.* 205, 65.

CONCLUDING REMARKS

By A. Lwoff, *Pasteur Institute, Paris, France*

AT THE ONSET of the nineteenth century, Pierre Bretonneau disentangled the doctrine of specificity of disease out of a terrific confusion of ideas and realized that the differences in the clinical and pathological pictures were due to differences in the nature of morbid causes. These were, later on, identified as microorganisms. A pathogenic microorganism is, by definition, the agent or potential agent of a disease, the disease being the reaction of the organism toward the pathogenic agent. And it is known that sometimes, specific substances produced by the microorganisms are responsible for specific symptoms or syndromes. But the active participation of the cells in the morbid process is of primary importance. It is in view of the existence of this participation that it may be useful to analyze the relations between infectious and noninfectious diseases and to see whether or not the borderline is as clear in nature as in textbooks.

Let me first call attention to the work performed in Paris for the past 20 years by J. Reilly and his group (1) which seems to have been overlooked in most countries. It has been shown, for example, by the Reilly school that a typical typhoidic syndrome can be produced in the rabbit by the injection of a few bacteria in the splanchnic ganglion. The same syndrome is observed when a small amount of toxin is deposited on the splanchnic nerve, or when the splanchnic nerve is submitted to an appropriate electrical or chemical stimulus. Here, the apparently specific enteric syndrome is the result of a reaction of the splanchnic ganglion. The bacteria produce a specific disease because of their enteric localization, which results in the toxin reaching the abdominal autonomic nervous system. The syndrome is not characteristic of the bacterial toxin but of the reaction of the nerve ganglion. The apparently specific disease, the enteric syndrome, the hemorrhages, the necrotic lesions, are not the result of a direct action of the bacterial toxins on the intestine but appear to be due to a specific reaction of a group of nerve cells to nonspecific stimuli.

It is important to know that the tissues and cells which, at first glance, appear to be the primary victims of a direct action of the toxin are, in fact, destroyed as a result of a "stimulation" of cells which may be

173

remote and whose active participation is essential for the establishment of the disease. A similar sort of conclusion can be derived from the study of the viral diseases of bacteria.

The idea that killing agents, such as X-rays or ultraviolet rays, kill the cells by destroying an essential structure has been accepted for a long time. This conception was quite natural because it was in harmony with prevailing concepts concerning death. It is easy and simple to visualize death as the result of the loss or alteration of a cellular structure or function. Nevertheless, because a theory is a generalization, the danger of a theoretical conception increases with the part of truth it contains. Biological theories, whether they deal with evolution, development, or disease, generally explain phenomena either in terms of the disappearance of an essential structure or organization, or in terms of the formation of a new structure. Our minds are tuned on what may be called a mode, either a negative or a positive mode. And it is apparently difficult to pass from one to the other, and, moreover, to realize that the two modes are not necessarily incompatible. Radiations sometimes kill because they destroy essential structures. Sometimes, however, radiations kill because they induce a gene to express its lethal potentiality. As revealed by the study of lysogenic and bacteriocinogenic bacteria, this potentitality may be the power to start a new synthesis (2). And this synthesis may sometimes result in the formation of virus particles.

We are used to thinking of viruses as pathogenic particles. That the multiplication of phage is a lethal process is in itself not surprising. But the notion that the synthesis of a nonviral material may also be fatal is quite recent, and may be important for the understanding of some cellular diseases.

In an induced lysogenic bacterium, the prophage enters the vegetative phase of its cycle, phage material is produced and multiplied, and bacteriophage particles are formed in practically all bacteria. It happens that some strains of inducible lysogenic bacteria are defective. When irradiated with an inducing dose of ultraviolet light they behave apparently just as a normal inducible lysogenic strain. The bacteria continue to grow for about 40 min and then they lyse. It happens that only a very small fraction of them produce phage, one over 10^5 to one over 10^7. However, all the bacteria die, obviously as the result of a disturbance which is identical with the phagic disease in its symptomatology and evolution. One could conceive of a condition in which the probability of the virus ever appearing would be infinitely small, that is to say practically absent. In fact, such a condition is known in the so-called bacteriocinogenic bacteria. These bacteria have the power to produce bacteriocins, such as colicins, which are, so far as we know, specific proteins. These proteins are able to kill sensitive bacteria of the same species. Normally, colicinogenic bacteria do not contain any detectable amounts of colicin. They perpetuate only the power to produce colicin. It was discovered that the synthesis of colicin may be induced by an irradiation with ultraviolet light or with organic peroxides. After irradiation, the colicin synthesis starts immediately and colicin accumulates inside the bacterium until it lyses, around the 70th minute. Thus, the production of colicin, which is a protein, is a lethal process.

All these systems which have been considered, normal lysogenic, defective lysogenic, bacteriocinogenic, perpetuate a genelike structure which is a potential lethal factor. When submitted to an appropriate stimulus, the balance of the system is upset and the potential lethal factor expresses its potentialities: syntheses are started which are, directly or indirectly, responsible for bacterial lysis. In lysogenic bacteria the phage particles are the end result of a bacterial disease; the prophage first, then the disease, and finally the virus. The important thing is that induced bacteria are killed, whether or not virus particles are produced. The virus particle is in this case an epiphenomenon—the result of a disease and not its cause.

It is perhaps necessary to recall that the two main characteristics of viruses, infectivity and pathogenicity, are never present simultaneously in a given phase. A temperate phage particle, for example, is infectious but not pathogenic. The prophage is not infectious and nonpathogenic. The only pathogenic phase is the vegetative phase which is devoid of infectivity. The common feature of these three phases is the genetic material which, being endowed with genetic continuity, must retain the same structure throughout the various phases—but exhibits widely different behavior according to the environment: it is inert in the virus particle, it behaves as a bacterial gene in the prophage state, and it is pathogenic during the vegetative phase.

For a long time the virus particle has dominated virology. We have been strangely submitted to the external appearance of things, and, in this respect at least, we were barbarians. We should be aware of the fact that the viral disease is characteristic only of one of the viral phases and that "viruses" should be regarded as concepts resulting from an integration of the various phases of the life cycle of an "abnormal" genetic material.

A sharp line of demarcation is generally drawn between infectious and noninfectious diseases. The study of the pathology of bacteria shows that this distinction is not always justified and that transitions exist between metabolic and infectious diseases—the common feature being a lethal synthesis controlled by a genelike structure which is a potential lethal factor.

Our symposium has now reached its end—and I have to close the discussion although I feel that many more problems could have been fruitfully discussed. It has been a successful meeting and the reading of the proceedings will certainly be stimulating. Many of us, I suppose, have reached a better understanding of the importance of the metabolism of the host and of the infectious agent in the disease process—and also of the interrelation between metabolic and infectious disease. My impression is that we all here are now firmly convinced of at least one thing, namely that the most interesting and important manifestation of life is disease. No disease, no physicians. No physicians, no Academy of Medicine, and who and what would we be?

It is now an agreeable duty for the chairman of this last session to thank the speakers on behalf of the organizers of the symposium, to thank the organizers of the symposium on behalf of the Academy of Medicine and to thank both the organizers of the symposium and the Academy of Medicine on behalf of the audience.

1. Reilly, J., Rivalier, E., Compagnon, A., Laplane, R., and duBuit, H. (1935). *Ann. Méd.* 37, 241.
2. A. Lwoff (1953). Bacteriol. Revs. 17, 269.

Author Index*

A

Abelson, P. H., 37, 38, 41, *43*
Abrams, A., 107, *115*
Adams, D. H., 45, 53, 54, 56, *59*
Adams, M. H., 119, *130,* 131, 140, 144, 148
Adelberg, E. A., *23*
Ajl, S. J., 38, 39, 42, *43*
Albaum, H. G., 106, *115*
Anderson, E. S., 134, *136*
Anderson, T. F., 117, 118, 120, *130*
Asselineau, J., 5, *23,* 159, *160*
Astbury, W. T., 4, *23*
Auerbach, V. H., 47, 49, 54, *59*

B

Bacon, G. A., 82, *83,* 110, *115*
Bail, O., 114, *115,* 160, *160*
Ball, E., 105, *116*
Bang, F. B., 99, *101*
Barker, H. A., 25, *33*
Bassani, B., 58, *59*
Bauer, D. J., 138, *147, 167, 169*
Bawden, F. C., 138, *147*
Beard, D., 164, 165, 166, *168, 169*
Beard, J. W., 164, 165, 166, *168, 169*
Becker, C., 96, *101*
Bender, A. E., 57, *59*
Bendich, A., 72, *76, 77*
Bentley, H. R., 151, *152*
Berger, L., 32, *34,* 143, *147*
Berger, R. E., 71, *76*
Bergmann, M., 145, *147*
Bertani, G., 133, *136*
Beutner, E. H., 18, *24*
Biesele, J. J., 71, *76*
Bigger, J. W., 83, *83*
Birmingham, M. K., 57, *60*
Bishop, G. H., 107, 115

Bissegger, A., 57, *60*
Blalock, A., 28, *33*
Bloch, H., 153, 154, 156, 157, 159, *160, 161*
Bloom, W. L., 102, 107, 114, *116,* 170, *172*
Boivin, A., 121, *130*
Bolton, E., 37, 38, 41, *43*
Bornstein, B. T., 25, *33*
Boyle, P. J., 66, 72, *78*
Braun, A. C., 111, *115, 116,* 151, *152*
Braun, W., 97, *101*
Bremmer, J. M., 5, *23*
Britten, R., 37, 38, 41, *43*
Brodie, A. F., 18, *24*
Broidy, B. A., 124, *130*
Bronfenbrenner, J. J., 107, *115, 116,* 118, *131*
Brooks, V. B., 108, *115*
Broquist, H. P., 67, 71, *76, 77*
Brown, D. H., 32, *34*
Brown, G. B., 72, 74, *76, 77*
Brown, L. M., 49, 56, 57, *59*
Bryson, V., 82, *83*
Buckle, G., 103, *116*
Bueding, E., 25, 26, 27, 28, 29, 30, 31, 32, *33, 34*
Burchenal, J. H., 66, 67, 70, 71, 72, 73, *76, 77, 78*
Burger, A. S., 107, *115*
Burgi, E., 72, *77*
Burmester, B. R., 165, *169*
Burn, J. H., 53, *60*
Burnet, F. M., 121, 126, 127, 129, *130*
Burrows, T. W., 82, *83,* 110, *115*
Burton, K., 38, 39, 41, *43*

C

Calvin, M., 4, 16, *23*
Campbell, J. E., 57, *59*
Campbell, P. N., 151, *152*
Canetti, G., 153, *161*
Carson, S. F., 38, 39, 42, *43*

---

*Numbers in italics indicate pages on which complete references appear.

177

Fling, M., 80, *83*
Foley, G. E., 71, *77, 78*
Folley, S. J., 48, 49, 54, *59*
Foster, J. W., 38, 39, 42, *43*
Fraenkel-Conrat, H., 49, 50, 54, *59*
Franklin, R., 110, *116*
Fraser, J. B., 63, *77*
Freeman, V. J., 134, *136*
Fruton, J. S., 145, *147, 148*
Furst, S. S., 72, *76*

G

Gale, E. F., 51, *59*
Garber, E. D., 110, *116*
Gard, S., 162, *163*
Garen, A., 118, *131*
Gäumann, E., 149, *152*
Gehrig, R. F., 37, 38, *44*
Geiger, J. W., 107, *115*
Gellhorn, A., 74, *78*
Geschwind, I. I., 49, 56, *60*
Gladstone, G. P., 107, 114, *116*
Goebel, W. F., 119, 122, *130, 131*
Gold, E., 156, *161*
Goldstein, A., 67, *77*
Goodwin, L. G., 69, *77*
Gordon, M. W., 52, *59*
Gottschalk, A., 126, 127, *130*
Grabar, P., 114, *116*
Graham, A. F., 119, *130*
Gray, C. T., 113, *116*
Green, I., 165, 166, *169*
Green, R., 96, *101*
Greenbaum, A. L., 48, 49, 54, *59*
Greenbaum, S. B., 75, *77, 78*
Greengard, H., 56, *59*
Gregg, G. W., 4, *23*
Grossberg, D. B., *116*
Grossman, M. I., 56, *59*
Gunnison, J. B., 82, *83*
Gunsalus, C. F., 19, *24*
Gunsalus, I. C., 19, *24*
Gurin, S., 41, *44*

H

Haas, V., 25, *33*
Hackett, A. J., 110, *116*
Hahnel, E., 12, *24*
Hakala, M., 75, *78*
Harden, A., 39, 40, *44*

Harper, E. M., 41, *44*
Harris-Smith, P. W., 114, *116,* 160, *161*
Harrison, H. C., 28, *33*
Harrison, M. F., 49, 56, 57, *59*
Hartman, P. E., 18, *24*
Hartree, E. F., *116*
Hawking, F., 68, 69, 71, *78*
Hawkins, J., 57, *59*
Hawthorne, H. R., 50, 58, *59*
Hayes, W., 5, *24*
Heagy, F. C., 120, 121, *130,* 133, *136*
Heckley, R. J., 114, *116*
Hendee, E. D., 104, *116*
Henderson, H. J., 18, *24*
Henion, W., 31, *34*
Henle, W., 123, 128, *130, 131*
Herriott, R. M., 120, *130,* 135, *136*
Hershey, A. D., 118, 119, *130, 131,* 134, *137,* 140, *147*
Hills, G. M., 37, *44*
Hirsch, J. G., 102, *116*
Hirshberg, E., 74, *78*
Hirst, G. K., 123, 124, 127, *131*
Hitchings, G. H., 68, 69, 71, 72, 73, 74, *76, 77, 78*
Hoagland, C. L., 167, *169*
Hoare, D. S., 7, *23*
Hobby, G. L., 82, *83*
Hodge, A. J., 4, *23*
Hogeboom, G. H., *24*
Holeman, D. F., 109, *116*
Holmes, W. L., 69, 74, 75, *77, 78*
Horne, R. W., 9, *24*
Horowitz, N. H., 80, *83*
Horsfall, F. L., 125, 126, 127, *131*
Hottle, G. A., 107, *115*
Houlahan, M. B., 7, *23*
Houwink, A. L., 4, 13, *23*
Hoyle, L., 125, 126, *131*
Huang, C. H., *147, 148*
Hughes, H. B., 71, *78*
Hunt, R., 57, *59*
Hutchison, D. J., 66, 67, 70, 71, *76, 77, 78*
Human, M. L., 133, *137*

I

Ingraham, J. L., 168, *169*
Isaacs, A., 125, 126, 127, 128, *130, 131*
Ivy, A. C., 56, *59*

J

Jackson, D. M., 111, *116*
Jacob, F., 134, 135, *137*, 138, *147*
Jambor, W. P., 156, *161*
Jawetz, E., 82, *83*
Jesaitis, M., 119, 122, *131*
Johnson, E. P., 164, *168*
Johnston, S. F., 66, *77*
Jones, M. E., 145, *148*
Jukes, T. H., 71, *77*
Jungherr, E., 164, *168*

K

Kabat, H., *148*
Kalmanson, G., 118, *131*
Kamen, M. D., 38, 39, 42, *43*
Karger, B., 75, *78*
Karnofsky, D. A., 71, 72, *77, 78*
Karzon, D. T., 99, *101*
Kegeles, G., 107, *113*, 114, *116*
Keilin, D., *116*
Kelner, A., 135, *137*
Kensler, C. L., 56, *59*
Keogh, E. V., 121, *130*
Keppie, J., 112, 114, *116*, 160, *161*
Kerr, L. M. H., 57, *59*
Kidder, G. W., 74, *78*
King, H. L., 51, 56, *59*
Kingsley-Pillers, E. M., 72, *77*
Kluyver, A. J., 3, *24*
Knaysi, G., 8, 18, *24*
Knight, B. C. J. G., 108, *116*
Knivett, V. A., 37, 38, *44*
Knoop, F., 42, *44*
Knox, W. E., 46, 47, 48, 49, 54, *59*
Kohler, A. R., 67, *76*
Kojima, Y., 104, *116*
Koletsky, S., 28, *33*
Koser, S. A., 41, *44*
Kozloff, L. M., 135, *137, 148*
Krampitz, L. O., 42, *44*
Kream, J., 74, *78*
Krebs, H. A., 35, 38, 39, 41, *43, 44*, 57, *59*
Kreps, E. M., 57, 58, *59*
Krimsky, I., 138, 142, 143, 144, *148*
Kuniati, K., 56, *59*
Kunitz, M., 32, *34*
Kurokawa, M., 104, *116*
Kushida, M. N., 66, *77*

L

Lamanna, C., 107, *116*
Lang, C. N. H., 28, *33*
Lanni, F., 124, *131*, 136, *137*
Lanni, Y. T., 124, 131, 135, 136, *137*
Laplane, R., 114, *116*
Lark, K. G., 119, *131*, 144, *148*
Laser, H., 27, *33*
Law, L. W., 66, 67, 72, *78*
Leach, R. H., 159, *161*
Leath, M. J., 53, *60*
Lecrone, B. L., 50, 58, *59*
Lederberg, S., 133, *137*
Lederer, E., 5, *23*, 159, *160, 161*
Lee, N. D., 47, 50, *59*
Leger, J., 58, *60*
Lehninger, A. L., 58, *60*
Leonard, C. S., 62, *78*
Leone, L. A., 72, *77*
Levine, S., 124, *131*
Levinthal, C., 136, *136*
Levvy, E. A., 57, *59*
Li, C. H., 49, 56, *60*
Liebl, G. J., 56, *59*
Lipmann, F., 167, *169*
Liu, C., 99, *101*
Liu, O. C., 128, *131*
Logan, M. A., 38, *44*
Lominski, I., 41, *44*
Long, C. N. H., 170, *172*
Lowbury, E. J. L., 111, 112, *115, 116*
Luria, S. E., 118, *131*, 133, 136, *136, 137*
Lurie, M. B., 153, *161*
Lush, D., 121, *130*
Lynch, V., 4, 16, *23*
Lwoff, A., 132, 133, 134, 135, *137*, 144, *148, 173, 174, 176*

M

Maas, W. K., 80, *83*
MacCallum, P., 103, *116*
McCarty, M., 13, 15, *24*
MacDonald, M., 32, *34*
McDermott, E. E., 151, *152*
McElroy, O. E., *116, 117*
Macfarlane, M. G., 108, *116, 167, 169*
Mackanness, G. B., 113, *116*
McKee, C. M., 156, *161*
Mac Kinnon, J., 28, 32, *33*
McKinney, 96, *101*

Subject Index

A

Acetic acid, microbial utilization, 41
  yeast oxidation, 41, 42
Acetoacetic acid, 39
Acetobacter suboxydans, 19, 22
Acetobacter xylinum, 8
Acetophosphokinase, 38
Acetyl-coenzyme A, 38
Acetyl phosphate, 38
Acidosis, 55
Acridine, 68
Actinomycetes, and diaminopimelic acid,
  5
Adaptation, 45
  and protein synthesis, 47
  parasite, host, 114
  substrate induced, 48
Adenine, 72
Adenosine deaminase, 52
Adenosinediphosphate, and citrulline, 38
  dephosphorylating enzyme, 166
  energy production, 36
Adenosinemonophosphate, and dephos-
  phorylating enzyme, 166
Adenosinetriphosphatase, and brain glycolysis, 143
  sodium fluoride, 172
  virus, 168
Adenosinetriphosphate, and brain metabolism, 143
  diphtheria toxin, 170
  Schistosome hexokinase, 32
  synthesis, 35, 36
  and citrulline, 38
  viral dephosphorylation, 164-168
  virus, 167, 168
Adenylic acid, see Adenosinemonophosphate
ADP, see Adenosinediphosphate.
Adrenal gland, tryptophan peroxidase
  adaptation, 48

Adrenocorticotropic hormone, 48
Adsorption, virus-enzyme, 167
Aerobacter aerogenes, 41
Age, and metabolic adaptation, 56, 57
Aggressin, 114
  and cord factor, 160
Alanine, and *Brucella mutation,* 97
D-Alanylglycine, 145
Alcaligenes faecalis, 171
Alcohol dehydrogenase, 171
Aldolase, 58
  iron containing, 88
Alkaline phosphatase, 52, 56
Alkalosis, 55
Alloxan diabetes, 96
Alumina Cγ, 32
Amidase, 127
Amine oxidase, 53
Amino acid, and bacterial cell wall, 10,
  11
  protein specificity, 8
  tularemia, 109
  derivatives, and brain glycolysis, 146
D-Amino acid oxidase, 56
  and adrenaline, 54
L-Amino acid oxidase, 55
α-Aminoadipic acid, 7
p-Aminobenzene-sulfonamide, 63
p-Aminobenzoic acid, 63
  and Malaria, 69
  sulfonamide inhibition, 81
α-Amino, ε-hydroxy caproic acid, 7
Aminopterin, 65-67
  and nucleic acid, 75
Aminoquinoline, 68
4-Amino-quinoline, 70
8-Amino-quinoline, 70
AMP, see Adenosinemonophosphate
Amylase, 56, 58
Anaerobiosis, and phage infection, 133
Anthrax, 108

BAL, see Dimercaprol
Basidiomycete, 6
Benzoylargininamide, 145
Blood, avian, and virus, 164
Blue-green algae, 4
  and diaminopimelic acid, 6, 7
  photosynthetic pigment, 4
  localization in cell, 15
Body fluid, metabolites, 96
Bond, energy, 35
Botulinus toxin, 107
Brain, glycolysis, 142, 143
  and iron, 144
  heat labile factor, 144, 145
  metabolism, 139
Brucella, 6
  mutation, 97
Brucella abortus, 98
Brucellosis, 98
Butyric acid, and *Ascaris,* 25
  fermentation, 40
Butyryl coenzyme A, 39

C

Canine hysteria, 151
Capsule, 8
Caproic acid, 25
Carbobenzoxyglycyllleucinamide, 145
Carbohydrate, and phage neutralization,
  122
  synthesis, 134
  metabolism, *Ascaris,* 26
  infected bacteria, 140, 141
  Schistosoma, 28
Carbonic anhydrase, 57
2-Carboxy pyrrole, 126
Carotenoid, 84
Catalase, 27
  and adrenaline, 54
Catechol, 86
Cathepsin III, 145
Cell structure, bacteria, 4
Cell wall, bacteria, 8-11
  ultrastructure, 13
  enzyme degradation, 11-13
  immunochemistry, 15
  isolation, 9
Cellulose, 9
Chemoautotrophy, 5

Chemotherapy, 43
  action mechanism, 79, 80
  and cancer, 74
  permeability, 89
  leukemia, 66
  sulfonamide, 81
Chitin, 9
Chlorella vulgaris, 111
Chloroguanide, 68
  resistance, 69, 70
Chloroplast, 4
  and Chromatophore, 16
Chloroquinone, 70
Chlorovinyl-dichloroarsine, 62
Choline oxidase, 57
Cholinesterase, 57
Chordata, 84
Chromosome, and bacteria, 5
  prophage, 133
Chromatophore, 15
  electron microscopy, 16, 17
Cilia, 4
Citric acid, and *Escherichia coli,* 41
Citric acid cycle, 36
Citrovorum factor, 66, 67
Citrulline, 37
Citrulline phosphate, 38
Clostridium botulinum, 107
Clostridium perfringens, aldolase, 88
  ornithine synthesis, 38
Clostridium tetani, and diaminopimelic
  acid, 5
  toxin, 107
Clostridium welchii, 109
Co I, see Coenzyme I
Co II, see Coenzyme II
Coenzyme I, 30
  and cytochrome b_5, 105, 106
    energy production, 36
    enzyme-antibody complex, 31
    glucose dehydrogenase, 88
  reduced oxidase, 171
  oxidation, 171
Coenzyme I-ase, 142
Coenzyme II, 29
  and direct glucose oxidation, 42
  glucose dehydrogenase, 88
Coenzyme A, 38
Coenzyme A transphorase, 39

SUBJECT INDEX

191

I

Immunity, and disease, 156, 157
Infection, and hypothermia, 170
  chronic, 153
  mechanism, 102, 103
Infectious hepatitis, 153
Inflammation, 96, 97
  and infection, 102
Influenza virus, adsorption, 124, 125
  and allantoic membrane, 125
    dinitrophenol, 168
    electrostatic forces, 129
    penetration, 125, 126
    morphology, 123
    red cell adsorption, 167
Intracellular receptor substance, 128
Iodoacetic acid, and bacterial lysis, 119, 120
Ion, and dephosphorylating enzyme, 166
  phage adsorption, 118
  and glyceraldehyde-3-phosphate dehydrogenase, 144
  toxin production, 107
Isobutyric acid, 25
Isoniazid, 157, 158

J

Janus green, 18

K

Kerateine, 62
2-Ketogluconic acid, 87
5-Ketogluconic acid, 87
α-Ketoglutaric acid, 36
Ketosis, and bacterial infection, 99
Klebsiella pneumoniae, purine requirements, 110
Knoop-Thunberg cycle, 42
Krebs-Henseleit cycle, 52
Kynurenic acid, 86
Kynureninase, 49
Kynurenine, 49

L

Lactic acid, and bacterial inhibition, 99
  mycobacteria, 102
  Schistosoma, 28
  fermentation, 39

formation by *Ascaris,* 25
Lactic acid dehydrogenase, 28
  Schistosome, 29
Lactobacillus bulgaricus, 75, 76
Lactobacillus casei, and folic acid, 67
  growth inhibition, 72
Lecithin, 108
Lecithinase, 108
Leprosy, 113
Leucinamide, 145
Leucine ethyl ester, 145
Leuconostoc citrovorum, 70
Leuconostoc mesenteroides, 7
Leucylglycine, 145
Leucylglycylglycylglycine, 145
Lichen, 84
Lipase, 58
Lipid, and *Ascaris,* 26
  bacterial cell wall, 8-10
Lipocarbohydrate, 122
Lipopolysaccharide, 86
Lipoprotein, 9
  and *Ascaris* succinoxidase, 27
Lobar pneumonia, 108
  symptoms, 109
Lycomarasmin, 110
  antagonist, 150
  chemistry, 149
Lysine, and diaminopimelic acid, 7
  microbial synthesis, 86
  lactic acid bacteria, 7, 8
Lysis, bacterial cell, 13, 14
  and adsorbed phage, 119, 120
  from without, 119-121
  protoplast, 14, 15
Lysogenic bacteria, and gene, 174
  induction, 174
Lysozyme, and cell wall studies, 11-13
  inhibition of activity, 13, 14

M

M antigen, 10
Malonic acid, 42
Malonamide, 145
L-Mandelic acid dehydrogenase, 19
Manganese, and *Ascaris* succinoxidase, 27
  Brucella mutation, 97
Mannokinase, 32
Mannose, phosphorylation, 32